*

RN's SEX Q&A

Candid Advice for You and Your Patients

Dorothy DeMoya, RN, MSN

Adjunct Clinical Assistant Professor
Catholic University of America School of Nursing
Washington, D.C.

Co-Director
Washington (D.C.) Reproductive Associates
Sexual Dysfunction Therapy Program

Armando DeMoya, MD

Clinical Assistant Professor of Obstetrics and Gynecology
Georgetown University Hospital and George Washington
University Hospital, Washington, D.C.

Co-Director
Washington (D.C.) Reproductive Associates
Sexual Dysfunction Therapy Program

Howard R. Lewis

Senior Associate Editor
RN Magazine

MEDICAL ECONOMICS BOOKS
Oradell, New Jersey 07649

Library of Congress Cataloging in Publication Data

DeMoya, Dorothy.
RN's sex Q & A.

Bibliography: p.
1. Sex instruction for the sick—Miscellanea.
2. Hospital patients—Sexual behavior—Miscellanea.
3. Nurse and patient—Miscellanea. I. DeMoya, Armando.
II. Lewis, Howard R. III. Title. IV. Title: R.N.'s
sex Q and A. [DNLM: 1. Sex—Nursing texts. 2. Sex
behavior—Nursing texts. WY 100 D388r]
HQ30.7.D45 1983 613.9'5'0880814 83-19299
ISBN 0-87489-360-7

Design by Douglas Steinbauer

ISBN 0-87489-360-7

Medical Economics Company Inc.
Oradell, New Jersey 07649

Printed in the United States of America

*

Dorothy and Armando DeMoya:
For Jerry, Don, and Rita

Howard R. Lewis:
For Eric and Carol

Contents

Preface

THIS BOOK is derived from the hundreds of questions that nurses and other health professionals have asked us through the SEX Q&A column of the nursing journal *RN*. This column originated in response to a need for down-to-earth advice on the most sensitive subjects in patient care.

These questions and answers deal not only with patient-care issues but also with readers' personal concerns. Before giving sexual information and advice to patients, health professionals need to be comfortable with their own sexuality.

Among other areas of broad practical interest to care givers, we seek to provide a better understanding of how diseases and other physical conditions may interact with sexual health. Throughout this book, we present findings from the new, multidisciplinary branch of health care called sexual medicine, which deals with how sexual activities can affect physical health and how medical conditions can influence sexual functioning. This new specialty draws on advances in gynecology, obstetrics, urology, pharmacology, endocrinology, psychiatry, and many other fields.

Many health professionals as well as patients are misled by a stereotype that equates sexuality with vigor—and thus decrees that the sexual urges of the aging, sick, or disabled are inappropriate or nonexistent. This leads many care givers and patients to assume that illness generally makes a satisfactory sex life impossible.

We are happy to help break down this misconception. A major part of this book offers information relevant to sexual functioning in specific impairments.

Medications are often administered without consideration of their influence on sexual functioning or reproductive capacity. We describe a wide variety of drugs and how they may affect sexuality.

Also covered in this book are the health effects of sexual activities. We deal with a large number of sexually transmitted diseases. We also discuss other types of genitourinary conditions, including injuries and anatomical problems. In addition, you'll find guidelines about contraceptive methods, covering their indications, effectiveness, and risks.

We'd like to extend our compliments and appreciation to the readers who've addressed important sexual issues in their personal and professional lives. We also are grateful to the scores of consultants who've offered comments and suggestions prior to publication.

We hope our efforts will expand health professionals' understanding of human sexuality and will promote greater sexual fulfillment for their patients and themselves.

Dorothy DeMoya, RN, MSN
Armando DeMoya, MD
Howard R. Lewis

bottom of page

Publisher's Notes

*

RN'S SEX Q&A: *Candid Advice for You and Your Patients* is based on material that first appeared in the popular SEX Q&A column in *RN Magazine.* In preparing this book, the authors expanded and revised their original answers and have grouped the material into such subject areas as: Sexual Attitudes and Behaviors; Sexual Response; Medical Conditions; Surgery-Related, Genitourinary, Obstetrical, and Gynecologic Problems; Menstruation and Menopause; Sexually Transmitted Diseases; Contraception; Fertility and Infertility; Masturbation; Homosexuality; Drugs and Sex; Sexual Dysfunction; and Problems in the Hospital.

Dorothy and Armando DeMoya, co-directors of the Washington (D.C.) Reproductive Associates Sexual Dysfunction Therapy Program, were the first sex-therapy team trained by Masters and Johnson in a pilot training program for professionals.

Dorothy DeMoya, RN, MSN, is adjunct clinical assistant professor and a doctoral student at the Catholic University of America School of Nursing. She taught human sexuality at Georgetown University School of Medicine and was secretary of the Society of Sex Therapy and Research.

Armando DeMoya, MD, is clinical assistant professor of obstetrics and gynecology at Georgetown University Hospital and George Washington University Hospital.

Howard R. Lewis, senior associate editor of *RN Magazine*, collaborates with the DeMoyas in producing the SEX Q&A column in that journal. He is also Q&A editor of *Sexuality and Disability*. Mr. Lewis and Martha E. Lewis are co-authors, with the DeMoyas, of *Sex and Health: A Practical Guide to Sexual Medicine* (Stein and Day, 1983).

Mr. Lewis has written extensively on a variety of medical subjects. His books include: *Sex Education Begins at Home, The Parent's Guide to Teenage Sex and Pregnancy, Psychosomatics: How Your Emotions Can Damage Your Health*, and *The People's Medical Manual: Your Practical Guide to Health and Safety*.

CHAPTER 1

*

Sexual Attitudes and Behaviors

*

YOU'RE LIKELY to encounter a host of sexual attitudes and behaviors among your patients, because the expressions of human sexuality are as wide-ranging and varied as the human imagination.

As an individual, you naturally have your own particular set of sexual preferences. You may be partial toward some types of sexual practice, possibly disapproving of others. As a health professional, however, you'll serve your patients best by being as nonjudgmental as possible. It's important to present patients with information, not moral postures.

We'd especially avoid imposing our own views of what's normal. When applied to sexuality, the word normal has little meaning statistically or clinically. Health professionals who work in areas of human sexuality generally accept as normal any mutually pleasurable act between consenting adults.

To explore your feelings about sexuality and be exposed to the ideas of others, you may wish to participate in a formal program designed to reassesss sexual attitudes. These are widely available through hospitals and medical schools.

* *Negative reactions to sight of sex organs*

I've observed that many patients are disgusted or frightened by the genitalia of the opposite sex. Doesn't this contribute to sexual dysfunction? Is there a remedy?

Anatomical misconceptions indeed often interfere with a couple's sexual functioning. We've seen women who feel about penises the way they feel about snakes, and men who have a notion that vaginas are laden with teeth. Many men and women also regard their own genitals as "dirty" or "ugly."

In our sex-therapy program, we seek to demystify the genitalia by performing conjoint physical exams, with each partner present throughout the other's checkup. We start out with a teaching session. Using models and pictures, we show them that "some women have a uterus that's anterior; others, posterior," and point out, "Here's the spermatic cord, attached to the testicle."

In the examining room, we position a mirror so that the woman can look through the speculum into her vagina. "Let's see if you have a posterior or anterior uterus," we say. If it's anterior, we help the woman feel it through her abdomen. Most couples are amazed to see the cervix, rugae, and other features. Similarly, we have the couple explore the man's testes and penis along with us.

This genital examination is part of a complete physical exam, which puts the sex organs in the context of the entire anatomy. Most couples leave with a better appreciation that the genitals are parts of the body like any other. One husband told us, "I used to be embarrassed over the thought of natural childbirth. Now it seems a whole lot more natural."

* *Frequency of intercourse*

A recently married young woman has asked about the normal frequency of intercourse among married couples. What should I tell her?

Such questions often mask patients' anxiety about their own practices. Most likely, your patient really wants to know whether her own rate is "normal." Reassure her that if she and her husband are in general agreement about their frequency of intercourse—whether it's once a day or once a year—there is no cause for concern. This is what is normal for them.

Also let her know that, at one time or another, almost every couple differ over how often they should have intercourse. Partners are unlikely to share identical levels of sexual desire, just as they're not likely to respond in exactly the same manner to hunger, fatigue, or joy. But the imbalance is rarely critical, and most couples can accommodate to it. Nor should they expect their frequency of intercourse to be consistent. Ebbs and flows are inevitable, often depending on such factors as health, job pressures, and the needs of their children.

* Fears about penis size

An adolescent boy worries that his penis is too small to satisfy a woman. On examination, it seems of normal size. How should I counsel him?

This is a common concern of normal teenage boys—and of many grown men as well. It stems from the myth that the larger a man's penis, the more sexual pleasure he gives women.

Reassure your patient that this is not true. Many men have an image of the vagina as a vault of a certain size that has to be filled by a sufficiently large penis. A much more accurate image is that of an elastic stocking or an empty sleeve. The vagina accommodates penises of varying sizes.

During sexual arousal, the opening of the vagina constricts, exerting a gripping force on the penis. At the same time, the inside of the vagina expands, decreasing direct stimulation from penile thrusting and making the size of the penis basically irrelevant. Further, the inner two-thirds of the vagina contains few sensory nerve endings, whereas there is a rich concentration of such nerve endings at the vaginal entrance.

Your patient may have observed in the locker room that his penis in its flaccid state is smaller than his friends' penises. Assure him that his *erect* penis is probably roughly the same size as theirs. Smaller flaccid penises usually double in size, and larger flaccid penises may increase only 80 percent. Thus the great variation in sizes of flaccid penises tends to even out when they're erect.

* Duration of foreplay

How much foreplay is recommended for the average couple?

Enough so that intromission is a pleasure, which usually means that the woman is adequately lubricated through sexual stimulation. This varies from couple to couple and from occasion to occasion. There's no average couple or fixed amount of time. The ideal is to do whatever feels good for as long as it's fun, treating lovemaking as a continuous episode of shared enjoyment.

"Foreplay" is, therefore, a misnomer. It implies that noncoital stages of lovemaking are but preliminaries building up to penetration, supposedly the main event. In fact, for women especially, sex play is often more pleasurable than is penile-vaginal thrusting. Indeed, containing the penis in the vagina may be merely one step in helping a woman become aroused to the point of orgasm.

* Penile entrapment: Can it happen?

Do people ever get stuck together during intercourse, or is that just a myth?

Penis captivus can occur but is extremely rare. Penile entrapment may result from the female's experiencing severe vaginismus during coitus. One physician reports relieving such a vaginal spasm by going to the couple's bedroom and putting the woman to sleep with a minimal IV injection of thiopental sodium (Pentothal).

See: Melody GF. A case of penis captivus. *Med Aspect Hum Sexuality* 11:111, Dec 1977.

* Sexual stirrings in a father

A father in his 30s fears he has incestuous longings for his eight-year-old daughter. When she sits on his lap he often gets an erection. Now he avoids this contact completely. What should I advise him?

Chances are his erection reflex is being triggered not by incestuous urges but by tactile stimulation. To avoid reflexive erections, all he need do is move the child to another part of his lap, where her movement won't stimulate the nerve endings in his genital area.

He ought to continue lap-sits, hugging, and other displays of affection for as long as his daughter—or son—welcomes them. Fathers often wrongly link their arousal to the child's sexual development. They push the youngster away, causing confusion and feelings of rejection ("What did I do wrong? Why is Daddy mad at me?").

Occasional fantasies about children of either sex are nearly universal among mothers and fathers. But, because these flickerings of the imagination are almost never discussed in public, they can make parents feel abnormal, frightened, and guilty. You can assure parents that any *fantasy* is OK, and that it's only taking action on one that could be damaging. Since their behavior controls are undoubtedly quite strong, there's little danger that they'll act their fantasies out.

* Intercourse-related vaginal sounds

When I have intercouse, air seems to rush out of my vagina, making embarrassing noises. What causes this? How can I prevent it?

It's likely that you're assuming coital positions in which your pelvis is elevated. Placing a pillow under your hips or lying supine with your knees close to your chest will do this. As a result, your uterus and posterior vaginal wall fall backward from gravity, causing a vacuum that sucks air through the vaginal opening. Changing your position can make the uterus and vaginal wall move, forcing air out. Penile thrusting, too, may introduce air into the vagina; the pistonlike motion may also force air out, contributing to the sounds.

These noises are perfectly normal. We would not recommend your trying to avoid them by abandoning coital positions you enjoy; an elevated pelvis tends to permit deep penile penetration, which is gratifying to many couples. Rather, we'd suggest that you accept these sounds as the background music of satisfying intercourse and explain them as such to your partner.

* *How to deal with teenagers and intercourse*

Do you ever discourage your teenage patients from engaging in sexual intercourse? Have you ever thought of saying, "If you're not ready for the commitment of marriage, you're not mature enough for intercourse"?

We suspect that behind your questions is a belief that we and other health professionals should discourage teenagers from intercourse because it belongs only in a marital relationship.

In fact, our personal feeling is that the best sexual expression exists within a monogamous, committed, loving relationship. But that's our private preference, and we have to remind ourselves that many people don't share it. Nor should they be expected to, given the myriad factors that shape every individual's sexual experience and perceptions.

We, therefore, try to avoid imposing our personal value system on patients. We feel we'd be invading their privacy—and taking advantage of our position—if we moralized to them. We tend to confine our recommendations to health-related matters and to give only asked-for advice.

We've found that teenagers, especially, tune out unsolicited sexual advice, and this can deprive them of valuable sources of needed information. Therefore, we neither encourage nor discourage teenagers to have intercourse, but we do try to show we're receptive to any sexual questions they have.

In taking a girl's history, we routinely ask, "Do you have bleeding between periods?" This leads to, "Do you experience bleeding after intercourse?" We follow this with, "Many young people have questions about sexual activity. Are there any questions you want answered?" If the girl wishes to pursue the subject, we're pleased to be of help; if not, we respect her privacy. She's likely to return if she feels the need for further discussion.

Sometimes a girl asks us, "Should I go to bed with my boyfriend?" That's usually a sign that she has unresolved conflicts. We make it clear that the decision is hers and that she has to take responsibility for it. We also point out that intercourse can raise problems that young people often can't anticipate. To help her make the choice that's right for her, we raise such questions as: Why does she want to have intercourse? What does she expect from it? To what extent, if any, is she feeling pressured? What's her understanding of the possible consequences? How will it affect her relationship with her boyfriend? Could she handle a breakup afterward? Have she and her boyfriend discussed these issues? Have they made plans for contraception?

Occasionally, a girl asks, "Is intercourse right before marriage?" We're prepared to explore the pros and cons with her, but if she's seeking a moral judgment, we reply, "That's a question of right or wrong, and we're not in a position to answer it." We suggest that the girl consult her parents, a clergy member, or some other mature, trusted person whose moral guidance can help her clarify her thoughts on the issue.

* *What to advise about vaginal exercise*

Is it true that vaginal exercise can increase a woman's sexual pleasure?

Very much so—and that of her partner as well. The pubococcygeal muscle, which incorporates the vaginal area, is rich in nerve endings. Toning up the muscle with the Kegel exercise increases its sensitivity during intercourse. A stronger muscle also enables the woman to grip her partner's penis tightly and squeeze rhythmically.

To teach the patient the exercise so that she's likely to do it, suggest that whenever she urinates she stop the flow two or three times for about three seconds each time. This provides the same effect as if she were bearing down on a penis.

This exercise is extremely valuable for postpartum patients. Not only does it build muscle tone for sexual pleasure, but it also, by improving circulation, reduces the pain and edema resulting from the episiotomy. We have patients start doing the exercise soon after delivery—indeed, in the delivery room if possible.

* *Is aural sex normal?*

A rather candid acquaintance of mine says she reaches orgasm after having her ear stimulated. Is this normal?

You're evidently describing a sensitive auriculogenital reflex. When the external auditory canal is gently stroked by a finger or tongue, Arnold's nerve (the auricular branch of the vagus nerve) is stimulated and can induce orgasm.

It's absolutely "normal" in the sense that it's consistent with generally healthy functioning. The more we learn about sexual behavior, the less we use such words as normal and abnormal to describe it. Statistically, the terms are meaningless; so little is known about human sexual functioning that no one can know how many people do what. Worse yet, in discussions of sexuality, people often unconsciously use the words normal to mean good and abnormal to mean bad.

To deal with sex objectively, it's generally helpful for health professionals to avoid such value judgments.

* *Advice for dealing with exhibitionists*

Today on the street I encountered an exhibitionist. I told him, "You'll catch cold." Can you suggest a better response?

On the street you're safest if you pointedly ignore an exhibitionist. Some men who expose themselves are potentially violent, so do nothing that could be interpreted as humiliating. If a man calls you over to his car, supposedly to ask directions—a ruse in about half of exposures—pretend that nothing out of the ordinary is happening.

You're wise to give a wide berth to an exposer who makes threatening gestures, shouts obscenities, or jumps out of a doorway. These are sadistic signs and may warrant calling the police. You also may wish to notify the police if you're pestered by an exposer—exhibitionists often expose themselves in the same manner time after time, and you may be on someone's "route." It's compassionate to remind the authorities of the psychological nature of the exhibitionistic act and to urge them to arrange for a psychiatric consultation before pressing charges.

If you see exhibitionists in a psychiatric setting, you'll find that the typical male patient is an otherwise responsible citizen: employed or in school, often married and a father, with an above-average education. He generally is passive and rigidly conventional. He's likely to be guilt-ridden over sex, suffering such problems as impotence and premature ejaculation. Often he's too frightened of women to make overtures to them in the normal way.

Even though the exhibitionist may have an erection and be masturbating, his motivation is primarily nonsexual—typically an expression of anger stifled since childhood. He perceives his bodily sensations of rage as sexual urges; so in response to a situation he finds frustrating or provoking, he may have a compulsion to expose his penis rather than directly express his hostility. What he seeks is an expression of shock or fear—or admiration that reassures him of his masculinity.

An exhibitionist who admits to his condition generally has an excellent prognosis in psychotherapy. Once he understands the relationship between his act of exposure and his feelings of anger, he can usually be taught better ways of expressing his hostility. His impulse to expose himself may remain, but he'll typically learn to control it.

* *Handling obscene phone callers*

What's the best way to deal with an obscene telephone caller? What motivates men to make such calls?

As soon as you realize that a call is obscene, hang up without saying another word. A total lack of reaction is usually the most discouraging response a caller can get. Resist the temptation to tell him off or bang down the receiver. That's just the kind of response that can prompt him to bother you again. If a caller is persistent, report the intrusion to your phone company, which can put a tracer on your line.

Many obscene calls are made by teenagers who derive a sense of mastery from offending propriety. Adult callers tend to be sexually insecure males, often too emotionally immature to make direct contact with women. Their various approaches generally place them in any of several categories: The "shocker" immediately pours out obscenities and threats, and is sexually stimulated by your fear and anger. The "seducer" plays Don Juan and may claim he's gotten your name from a friend. After you've dropped your guard, perhaps even expecting him to ask for a date, he interjects obscene words and suggestions. The "surveyor" is a telephonic Peeping Tom who tries to get you to reveal sexual details about yourself by pretending to be a professional conducting a Kinsey-type study.

The fact that you're a nurse may attract such men, but you have absolutely no professional responsibility toward them. It's extremely rare for an obscene caller, even one who makes threats, to be violent or dangerous. Still, it's never safe to lead one on or accept a date.

* *Diseases from cunnilingus*

What diseases can be spread during cunnilingus? Are there microorganisms normal to the mouth that can cause vaginal infection, or, vice versa?

If an organism is nonpathogenic to either the oral or the vaginal mucosa, it usually won't cause problems if transmitted during cunnilingus. Conversely, pathogenic flora present in one mucosa may cause infection in the other.

Thus gonorrhea, syphilis, lymphogranuloma venereum, herpes simplex, and cytomegalovirus infections may be passed back and forth during cunnilingus. Any form of vaginitis—whether from *Trichomonas, Candida,* or bacteria—can lead to a corresponding mouth lesion.

From the oral cavity, the pathogens causing gingivitis or a tooth abscess may result in a comparable vaginal infection. Likewise, a strep throat or staphylococcal glossitis may give rise to bacterial vaginitis. We've seen some women develop vulvar inflammations as a result of allergies to their sex partners' lipstick and other cosmetics. And, in theory at least, antiseptic mouthwashes can reduce the vaginal bacterial count and allow a pathogenic overgrowth of other organisms.

* *Palatable contraceptive creams*

Is cunnilingus safe for the male after the woman has inserted contraceptive cream? Can you recommend any creams that taste good?

Contraceptive cream is nontoxic even if ingested orally. We know of no brand that's especially pleasant to the tastebuds. Many of our patients find contraceptive jelly (also safe) to be somewhat more palatable; it's faintly minty.

We're asked these questions so often that we wish more contraceptive manufacturers would face up to the realities of oral sex and add a really effective flavoring to their spermicidal barriers.

* *Soft palate injury from fellatio*

My 19-year-old niece has a band of ecchymoses and petechiae in the back of her mouth. She's asked me in confidence if this can result from engaging in fellatio with her boyfriend. What can I tell her? What treatment is needed?

The lesion you're describing can indeed result from fellatio. Negative pressure combined with elevating and tension of the soft palate can cause interstitial hemorrhage in this richly vascular area. Blunt trauma to the palate from vigorous fellatio can contribute to the submucosal injury.

You can assure your niece that the lesion is benign and usually heals in less than 10 days. You also might remind her that this is one of the forms of sexual activity that can transmit venereal disease, an argument for being prudent in choosing a sex partner.

In taking the history of a patient with palatal bruising, it may be reasonable to inquire discreetly if he or she engages in oral intercourse. By promptly considering fellatio as the origin, you may spare the patient workups for systemic causes that include infectious mononucleosis, nasopharyngeal tumor, and blood dyscrasias. Such injuries may also arise from playing a wind instrument, from impact with an object such as a straw or ice cream stick, or from violent spasms of coughing, sneezing, or vomiting.

See: Bellizi R, Krakow AM, and Plack W. Soft palate trauma associated with fellatio: Case report. *Milit Med* 145:787, 1980.

* *Reactions to swallowing semen*

What are the risks in swallowing semen? A woman complains of nausea and vertigo after ingesting her husband's ejaculate. She thinks she may be allergic to testosterone.

If the semen were contaminated, it could cause gonorrheal pharyngitis or syphilis of the oral pharynx. Viral disease, including herpes simplex and cytomegalovirus infections, can also be transmitted this way.

Otherwise semen is aseptic. We know of no case of its causing a food-type hypersensitivity. And you can tell your patient that testosterone is not a constituent of semen; the hormone is secreted directly into the bloodstream.

More likely, your patient's reaction is psychogenic. It's not unusual for a woman to enjoy fellatio but still have an aversion to her partner's ejaculating in her mouth. Although she may permit it, fearing that refusal will upset him, she may nevertheless feel used. This emotional conflict can be manifested physically in several ways; including nausea, vomiting, headache, and vertigo.

It might help to explore with your patient the reasons she's reluctant to tell her partner about her aversion. Role-playing such a confrontation could help her assert her wish that he withdraw before ejaculation.

* *Fear of urination during sex*

Several young women who are engaging in sexual relations for the first time have asked me if a man can urinate during ejaculation. I'm fairly sure there's a sphincter controlling the elimination of urine from the bladder during climax, but I'm not sure of the physiological mechanism. This is a particularly important question for those who are having oral sex and fear that a partner may void in their mouths.

You can reassure these young women that an erection engorges the prostate gland, closing off the prostatic portion of the urethra. This mechanism is not really a sphincter (it's not a muscle); nonetheless, it blocks the bladder so that urination is extremely unlikely to occur while the male is sexually aroused.

You might also explore with them whether they're uncomfortable with their degree of sexual involvement, especially if they seem troubled or confused. An inexperienced young woman's image of a partner urinating in her mouth could represent a number of negative feelings: She might have reservations about her relationship, feel unsure of what's being expected of her, or not know how to communicate her desires, and thus may feel pressured into sexual activity beyond her point of readiness. She also might have anxieties over oral-genital contact and interpret it as a form of humiliation. Indeed, she may be uninformed about many areas of sexuality. Your discussing such issues could do much to clear up problems.

* *Oral sex and cold sores*

Does the presence of a cold sore on the lip rule out performing fellatio or cunnilingus?

Definitely. *Any* lesion on the mouth should rule out oral sex. Otherwise, the infection may be transmitted from one partner to the other.

There's a myth that herpes simplex can't be spread through oral sex because, supposedly, the oral and genital viruses are different. True, type I *Herpesvirus hominis* most often affects the oral cavity, causing cold sores. But it can nonetheless cause painful lesions on the genital mucosa and create grave obstetrical hazards. Conversely, type II—the most frequent cause of herpes genitalis—can infect the lips, mouth, and tongue.

* *Infections from anal sex*

What are the dangers of infection from anal coitus? How can they be avoided?

In men, fecal contamination may result in urethritis. In women, rectal flora may be transferred to the vagina and urethra via the partner's contaminated penis. Coliforms present the major danger; *Salmonella* and *Shigella* organisms also may be transferred this way.

It's advisable to use a condom during anal coitus, expecially if the anal penetration is to precede vaginal intromission. As an alternative, you might recommend having vaginal coitus before anal—there's little danger of normal vaginal flora infecting the rectum. At the minimum, the male partner should urinate and wash his penis with soap and water as soon as possible after anal penetration, certainly before entering the vagina.

Gonorrhea, syphilis, and other venereal diseases can also be transferred through anal intercourse. Any patient with a sexually transmissible disease thus needs an anorectal smear. Anal warts are a frequent problem in people who receive anal coitus and recipient men have an elevated rate of bacterial prostatitis.

* *Anal fissures from intercourse*

Several of my patients have anal fissures as a result of anal intromission. How are they treated? Avoided?

Most of these linear, ulcerated lacerations of the anal canal are superficial and heal within three weeks with conservative measures. A stool softener and low-residue diet can ease the stretching of the anus during defecation, a cause of extreme pain and spasm. Before and after bowel movements, the introduction of lidocaine (Xylocaine) or another anesthetic ointment into the anal canal can also reduce pain. Spasms can be relieved by a sitz bath immediately after defecation. If a fissure becomes chronic, it may require surgical excision, with removal of the sentinel pile, the edematous skin tag that's often present at the lower end of the fissure.

Fissures are the most common injury from anal intromission. To prevent them, warn patients to engage in anal intercourse only if the receiving partner is willing and ready. When the recipient enjoys it and is relaxed, the sphincter usually dilates fairly easily. Insertion is then essentially painless and, indeed, can be pleasurable because of the anus's rich supply of nerve endings. Conversely, if the recipient submits only to please the partner, there is likely to be sphincter tightening, difficult penetration, and considerable trauma.

Injury may be avoided with gentle penetration and the use of a lubricant such as surgical jelly, a hypoallergenic oil, or a lubricated condom. Insertion is also eased if the receiving partner has defecated, emptying the rectum. Stroking the sphincter can help relax it.

Caution patients against anal coitus in the presence of a fissure or any other injury or any disorder such as hemorrhoids, fistula, stricture, or proctitis. Fissures also may result from anal tuberculosis or carcinoma. Examination is easiest with the patient in the knee-chest position; after a fissure is treated, sigmoidoscopy is advisable to rule out underlying disease. Recurring fissures are a signal for the patient to seek other modes of sexual expression.

* *Does anal sex cause homosexuality?*

I was brought up in the old school and don't seem to know different ways of enjoying sex. My husband used his mouth on my anus. I yelled at him that I didn't like it, and he hasn't touched me since. I think he is trying to make a homo out of me. What kick do people get out of that? Was I wrong in saying so to my husband?

Anolingual caress is a form of sexual expression widely practiced among heterosexuals as well as homosexuals. Whether you enjoy it or not is a matter of personal choice; the anus is richly endowed with nerve endings that have an erogenous potential, but many people are uncomfortable about anal stimulation often because they have negative feelings about the excretory system.

Further, there's a widespread myth that anal sex causes homosexuality; in fact, no one knows all the factors that account for sexual orientation, but it's clear that no sexual activity can make a heterosexual into a homosexual or vice versa.

You certainly have a right to express your sexual preferences; indeed, your husband would have done well to first ask you if you'd enjoy this form of sexual activity. However, yelling at your husband during love making may have left him feeling rejected and angry, as is suggested by his behavior toward you. We suspect that both of you could readily resolve your conflicts if you frankly explored the subject of sexual options.

CHAPTER 2

*

Sexual Response

*

HUMAN BEINGS are born with the capacity to respond sexually—to achieve erection, lubricate vaginally, have orgasms, and so on.

The awareness that sexual response is a natural, genetically determined physical phenomenon is one of the most significant contributions that Masters and Johnson have made to the study of human sexuality. It puts to rest psychoanalytic opinion that sexual response is learned behavior.

What *is* learned is sexual behavior: how one deals with one's sexual response. In this chapter, we chiefly address questions raised in connection with the orgasmic response.

* *Orgasm: Clitoral vs. vaginal*

What is the difference between vaginal and clitoral orgasm? Does having a D&C affect the ability to have either type?

An orgasm is an orgasm is an orgasm. There's only one type. It's a whole-body response and it can be achieved in many ways: through vaginal intercourse, oral stimulation, breast stimulation, clitoral stimulation, etc. Unfortunately, many women feel they are sexually inadequate because they can't achieve what Sigmund Freud called a "mature" vaginal orgasm as opposed to an "immature" clitoral orgasm.

Freud was inaccurate in postulating two kinds of orgasm in women. The clitoral orgasm is supposedly achieved when the clitoris is directly stimulated during masturbation, petting, and intercourse. This, Freud said, is an immature kind of orgasm, related to childhood sexual experiences. Freud considered the mature, ultimate sexual experience for a woman to be vaginal orgasm—which he thought occurred only in coitus, through the movement of the penis in and out of the vagina.

In fact, this is a male fantasy. Most men achieve orgasm during intromission—and erroneously assume that women must climax in the same way. A women often needs to inform her partner that the mere thrusting of his penis is not enough to lead her to orgasm. For her, intromission may be but one pleasurable stage of lovemaking. To reach orgasm, she may require additional stimulation, of whatever sort she finds gratifying.

Physiologically, a D&C does not affect a woman's ability to achieve orgasm. However, some women suffer a psychological reaction to this procedure. You may avert such problems by reassuring D&C patients that their genitalia are not damaged and that they are in no way diminished as women.

* *Are orgasms needed for a woman's health?*

One of my patients wants to know if orgasms are necessary for her physical health. How should I answer her?

You can tell her that even a lifelong absence of sexual arousal is in no way deleterious to one's health. Physiologically, an orgasm is the sudden relief of the pelvic vasocongestion that occurs with sexual stimulation. If that stimulation does not arise, there's no sex-induced engorgement—and no physical need for orgasm.

However, your patient may be hinting at another problem. If a woman repeatedly experiences sexual arousal but fails to reach orgasm, she may develop the pelvic congestion syndrome. Her symptoms are most likely to be pelvic discomfort and backache. These are usually accompanied by dysmenorrhea, an increased menstrual flow, and a watery vaginal discharge.The heavy aching distress is likely to make her extremely irritable. This is a relatively common condition, although women rarely link it to their sexual frustration.

On examination, there's generally diffuse tenderness when the lower abdomen is palpated. Vulvar tissues are swollen and sensitive. The vagina may go into spasm when touched. The vaginal mucosa is likely to be dark and soft, as in pregnancy. The uterus is probably tender.

The treatment is release of sexual tension. Advise your patient to explore what gives her pleasure—and tell her to share this information with her partner. Remind her, too, that she need not rely on her partner to bring her to orgasm.

* Female sexual response time

A woman complains that her husband gets impatient over her delay in reaching orgasm. Is there a drug or technique that you can recommend to speed her up?

On the contrary, we'd advise both partners to quit hurrying and accept the physiological differences that typify male and female sexual response times. Psychiatrist Domeena C. Renshaw of Loyola (Chicago) University's Stritch School of Medicine reports that a woman's response cycle, from arousal through orgasm, usually lasts about 13 minutes. By contrast, a man's cycle takes an average of only 2.8 minutes, barely long enough for most women to achieve vaginal lubrication. To avoid the suggestion that these are magic numbers that set some kind of norm or standard, we'd hasten to add that some women take much less time and some men take much more—sexual response is highly individual.

Counseling may help your patient avert sexual dysfunction. Because a mere 20 to 30 percent of women reach orgasm through coitus, many mistakenly conclude they are deficient and lose interest in sex. You might explain to both husband and wife that most women require more extensive sex play than men, including direct stimulation of erogenous areas. If the wife communicates what she'd like him to do, and if he slows down to her timetable, they both can enjoy sex in a leisurely fashion.

See: Renshaw DC. Is it orgasmic dysfunction or just bad timing? *Mod Med* 48:29, Dec 15.

* Vaginal lubricants

What lubricant would you recommend for relief of dyspareunia? I've heard many women patients complain of dry vaginal mucosa causing painful intercourse.

The ideal lubricant is the woman's natural moisture. Its absence suggests that your patients are experiencing intromission without being sexually aroused.

The first indication of a female's sexual arousal is a vaginal "sweating reaction": Vasocongestion causes fluid to seep from the smaller blood vessels, creating a film of droplets on the vaginal wall. In most instances, a woman more easily reaches orgasm if she first passes through this earlier phase of her sexual response cycle. Thus, external lubrication may relieve her vaginal dryness—but won't enable her to achieve orgasm without other arousal.

The most frequent cause of dyspareunia is the woman's failure to let her partner know what she finds sexually stimulating. It's often helpful to remind patients, both male and female, that they are responsible for their own sexual pleasure—and that their partners aren't mind readers.

Counsel patients to *express* what they want stroked, kissed, played with and how softly, slowly, or whatever. Encourage them to explore what they find most arousing; and remind them that they also need to say right out what they find displeasing. This process puts them in communication not only with their partners but also with their own bodies.

Adequate stimulation will usually relieve vaginal dryness. If additional lubrication is needed, saliva may be sufficient. Water-soluble contraceptive or surgical jelly is also effective. Postpartum women especially may need additional lubrication. Lactogenic hormones tend to cause a temporary decline in steroid output that decreases vaginal transudation.

Advise patients *against* using petroleum jelly as a lubricant. It obstructs natural vaginal lubricants and can impede the vagina's self-cleansing mechanism. Moreover, if the male wears a condom, a petroleum product could damage the thin rubber.

Also recommend against using cold cream as a lubricant. Many creams are mixed with oils and they often contain perfumes that can cause a vaginal allergic reaction.

* Not one orgasm in 46 years

In all my 46 years of married life I have never had an orgasm. I would not even know what to expect. The only suggestion I can offer is that I fell astraddle on an iron railing when I was about 11, which caused my crotch to hurt for perhaps an hour.

Could that have dislocated something? My husband wants me to enjoy sex with him, but there is nothing I can do. I could never ask a doctor for advice for fear he would misunderstand.

Good for you for recognizing that aging need not be a barrier to sexual enjoyment! The fact that you've been married for 46 years suggests that you are at least in your mid-60s. We wish it were more widely appreciated that older people can and do find sexual satisfaction.

However, we don't agree with some other assumptions you express. For one thing, it's unlikely that any competent, reasonably sensitive physician would "misunderstand" if you asked him for advice. Sexual dysfunction is a common symptom of many conditions. The first step in treating orgasmic dysfunction is a physical exam to rule out illness, injury, adverse drug reactions, and other physiological causes.

It's also extremely unlikely that an injury of the sort you describe so damaged your genitals as to render you incapable of having an orgasm. Even a woman whose clitoris—a richly innervated region—has been removed can ordinarily experience sexual gratification.

Most often, orgasmic dysfunction is a product of the sexual relationship —and here we disagree that there is "nothing" you can do. Indeed, a stereotypically "feminine" passive response is a major contributor to many women's difficulties in experiencing orgasm. If you're like such women, you need to take responsibility for your own sexual pleasure.

How well do you communicate with your husband what you like and dislike in sex? What gives each person pleasure is highly individual, and any form of sexual stimulation between consenting adults is perfectly fine as long as it's not done at the expense of the other person. Since few people are gifted with ESP, most need to be told explicitly what sex partners enjoy. The discovery of areas of sexual pleasure and the further exploration of them usually lead to orgasm.

You're likely to find that you'll need stimulation before, during, and after intromission in order to reach a climax. We've seen many women who don't reach orgasm during coitus and then give up on themselves as frigid. In fact, the Great Intercourse Myth cannot be exploded too often: Most women do *not* experience orgasm from penile thrusting alone. While it may be great fun, especially for the man, it often does not provide enough stimulation of the clitoris and other female erogenous areas to bring about orgasm.

In addition, to what extent are you *striving* for orgasm? Nothing is more fatal to reaching a climax than anxiety over achieving it, a common problem for task-oriented people. We often advise patients to put orgasm on a back burner—and, instead, go for what they enjoy doing. Orgasms come most readily when they matter least. If you adopt the attitude, "If I don't, I don't," then we wouldn't be surprised if you do.

* *Simultaneous orgasms*

I've always understood that a simultaneous orgasm is the highest goal in lovemaking, but my boyfriend doesn't agree. What do you say?

We agree with your boyfriend. If simultaneous orgasms happen by accident, wonderful. Otherwise, we'd say, forget them. Far from being a sign of superior sexual achievement, the effort to "come together" can ruin sex.

Striving to coordinate such basically involuntary responses can cause the partners to observe themselves ("Should I wait? Hurry up? Am I too slow? Too fast?")—a sharp contrast to immersing themselves in the pleasures of lovemaking. Such a spectator role can lead to impotence and orgasmic dysfunction. What's more, if simultaneity *is* achieved, it can deprive each partner of a possibly greater pleasure: observing, without distraction, the other's orgasm.

In general, the most satisfying lovemaking is an unself-conscious process. If you tune in to your body, moment by moment it's likely to signal what will feel good, often culminating in orgasm. A "goal" superimposed by the mind tends to thwart the process.

* *How to counsel a woman who fakes orgasm*

A young woman, frustrated by her boyfriend's inability to bring her to orgasm, has asked me how she might communicate to him her desire for oral and manual stimulation of her vulva, which she's found effective in previous relationships. She's afraid of being rejected by this man and also of seeming "too experienced" (which he's teased her about). She cares deeply for him, and sometimes fakes an orgasm to please him. What do you advise?

If this relationship is to continue with mutual satisfaction, we'd suggest that your patient trust her boyfriend enough to tell him what pleases *her*. She can help him along by providing lots of positive reinforcement ("That feels good!"); otherwise, how's he supposed to know? Indeed, everyone's sexual response is unique and varies from one time to the next, so partners constantly need to learn anew how they can please each other.

You also might discuss with the young woman what her boyfriend's teasing her about being "too experienced" could mean. Teasing is often hostile, and he may feel threatened by her sexual relationships with previous men (how does he compare to them? what kind of woman is she, anyway?).

Faking an orgasm is generally a bad idea: It's rarely convincing; it merely perpetuates the problem; and it puts an exaggerated emphasis on the goal of the orgasm rather than the pleasure of the process. Your patient, her boyfriend, and their relationship would be best off if she assumed responsibility for her sexual gratification and asserted her sexual needs.

* *Appearance of rash during sex*

A patient is concerned because she often breaks out in a rash during intercourse. It goes away following orgasm. Can you offer an explanation?

You're apparently describing the "sex flush," a measles-like erythema that often results from superficial vasocongestion. Late in the excitement phase or early in the plateau phase of the sexual response cycle, there can be a prominent dilation of the capillaries in the epigastrium, breasts, and chest wall. The reddening may spread to the buttocks, back, extremities, and face.

While the rash can be alarming, especially in fair-skinned people, you can tell your patient that it's perfectly normal, occurring in 50 to 75 percent of women and a smaller percentage of men. With aging, it tends to appear less frequently, with more limited distribution over the body.

CHAPTER 3

*

Medical Conditions

*

A MEDICAL condition, especially if it's chronic, is bound to have impact on your patient's sexuality.

The relationship between illness and sexuality varies considerably from person to person, depending on the nature and severity of the medical problem and the patient's age, personality, social circumstances, and previous sexual adjustments.

In some cases, the illness causes changes that directly impair the physiology of sexual response. This is true, for example, in multiple sclerosis, spinal cord injury, and other disorders of the central nervous system. Hormonal changes that affect libido similarly impair sexual functioning in a direct manner. Any illness that interferes with vascular supply to the pelvis, such as Leriche's syndrome, also directly impedes sexual functioning.

You need your sharpest clinical sense, however, for illnesses that *in*directly affect sexuality. Any condition that produces pain, weakness, or fatigue is likely to reduce sexual interest and activity. A person with heart or lung disease may be unable to tolerate the increased oxygen demands of intercourse. Chronic dermatological conditions can make sexual contact uncomfortable.

To elicit a patient's sexual concerns or problems, you might start by asking nonthreatening physiological questions such as "How has your menstrual period been affected?" or "Do you have any problem with urination?" These can lead the way to questions about changes in sexual desire or orgasmic or erectile difficulties.

You might further ascertain the patient's reaction to the illness. Depression or anxiety about the condition will usually interfere with sexual functioning. Assess the sex partner's attitude as well. A patient whose partner is anxious or repelled is likely to avoid sexual activity.

Also determine if medications or concurrent illnesses may be contributing to sexual impairment.

You can suggest that patients engage in sexual activity when they're well rested. If intercourse is difficult or impossible, other modes of sexual expression may be acceptable.

* *Rule of thumb for post-MI intercourse*

Many of my post-MI patients fear they'll have another heart attack if they resume intercourse. Is there a rule of thumb I can give them so they can tell if they're physically ready?

Yes. You can tell them they almost certainly can handle the cardiovascular challenge of intercourse if they can walk for 10 minutes at the rapid rate of 120 paces per minute and then climb two flights of steps in 10 seconds at a rate of two steps per second.

See: Larson JL, McNaughton MW, Kennedy JW, et al: Heart rate and blood pressure responses to sexual activity and a stair-climbing test. *Heart Lung* 9:1025, 1980.

* *Sex after heart attack*

What counseling should I give post-MI patients about resuming sexual activity?

Good question! Masters and Johnson found that two-thirds of patients who had suffered myocardial infarction were given no sexual advice at all during their medical treatment. The advice given the remaining third was so vague as to be useless.

Out of fear of precipitating another heart attack, many patients abstain from sex—causing frustration and marital conflicts that may make their cardiac condition worse. The patient's spouse or other sex partner often shares this anxiety. It's therefore important that both partners receive counseling.

You can tell them that the less-taxing forms of sexual activity are a good beginning; they boost confidence and ease the resumption of intercourse. Encourage the couple to engage in pleasuring (touching, cuddling, stroking) when the patient returns home. This kind of gentle activity, particularly when it's done without expectation of intercourse, helps relieve anxieties that can result in impotence.

Your patient can safely go on to masturbation or oral sex as soon as he can tolerate an accelerated heart rate of 130 beats per minute. In an uncomplicated recovery, this usually occurs after four to eight weeks.

You can also reassure your patient that intercourse takes much less effort than is popularly believed—and that heart attacks during intercourse are extremely rare. In fact, fighting a traffic jam or having an argument can be more stressful—and more dangerous. Your patient can usually resume intercourse when he's able to climb two flights of stairs or walk several blocks at a brisk pace. On objective tests, this equals exercise at levels of 6 to 8 cal/min. The average patient achieves this about 16 weeks post-MI.

The best time for intercourse is in the morning after a restful night's sleep. Three positions that lessen cardiac workload are recommended for the postcoronary patient. These are lying on the side, in a face-to-face position; lying on the back, with the partner on top; and for men, sitting on a wide chair, low enough for the feet to touch the ground.

Your patient will be under least physiological stress if the room is reasonably cool. Hot, humid weather—and unaccustomed high altitudes—can make intercourse risky. It's similarly advisable for your patient to refrain from having intercourse for three hours after eating a heavy meal or drinking alcohol.

Remind patients that sex with a new partner can be extremely taxing. Patients in these circumstances are likely to be under emotional stress from guilt, unfamiliar surroundings, and anxiety over performing. In addition, such an encounter usually follows an evening of heavy eating and drinking.

It's important to caution your patient to stop his activity if angina occurs during intercourse and to report the incident—and any angina that occurs *after* intercourse. He may merely need to use nitroglycerin prophylactically, taking it just prior to intercourse. Also urge your patient to report other danger signs: palpitation that continues for 15 minutes or more after intercourse, sleeplessness caused by sexual exertion, or marked fatigue on the day after intercourse.

If your patient's sexual rehabilitation is not succeeding, suspect depression. His emotional reaction to his heart attack may be impairing his sexual function, and additional counseling may be in order.

* Sex and a cardiac pacemaker

What sexual counseling is advisable following implantation of a cardiac pacemaker?

You might caution the patient to limit physical activity for the first two weeks after the pacemaker is implanted. This will permit adequate healing of the wound and avoid dehiscence that could lead to infection and pacemaker malfunction. This general limitation would make active intercourse inadvisable but wouldn't necessarily rule out masturbation or other nonstrenuous forms of sexual activity. Indeed, beginning such low-demand activities as soon as possible promotes sexual rehabilitation.

When recovery is complete, the patient may engage in any sexual activity that's comfortable. You can reassure patients that the pacemaker itself necessitates no restrictions whatever. It won't break or shake loose during coitus. Nor will close proximity to it cause harm to the partner from "radiation." If the disease process continues to make the patient too tired for sex, despite his desire, you might suggest having intercourse in the morning or after a rest.

* *Finding an antidysrhythmic that won't cause impotence*

To combat tachycardia and dysrhythmias, my husband first received disopyramide phosphate (Norpace), but it caused urinary retention. Then a switch to quinidine sulfate (Quinidex, Quinora) gave him a body rash. Now procainamide HCl (Procan, Pronestyl) is making him impotent. Is there any other drug he might take?

Very possibly. A cardiologist who's alert to such sexual side effects generally tries different medications and adjusts dosages until the dysrhythmia is controlled without significant adverse reactions, including impotence. We'd suggest that you and your husband have a frank talk with his cardiologist to make sure that the doctor takes impotence seriously; we've met cardiologists who'd give up on your husband, believing he should be satisfied because impotence is his only problem.

* *Intercourse and the hypertensive patient*

Since intercourse raises blood pressure, is it contraindicated for patients suffering from hypertension? Will decreased sexual activity lower blood pressure?

No on both counts. While blood pressure is normally elevated during the sexual response cycle, the effect is only transient and has nothing to do with cardiovascular hypertensive disease. Similarly, abstinence has no bearing on the mechanism that controls blood pressure. If anything, it can be argued that sexual activity in moderation can be helpful for hypertension because it decreases tension.

* *How to ask about impotence from antihypertensives*

What's the best way to ask if a patient on antihypertensive drugs is suffering the common side effect of impotence?

You might build up to it with questions about general sluggishness—at work, sports, other activities. It's not too hard to move from that to questions about sluggishness in the patient's sexual response, and that gives you an opening to explore how this makes him and his partner feel and to point out that this is, indeed, a common problem that can be overcome.

Often a man used to a rapid response panics. He either becomes psychogenically impotent, or stops taking the medication. It may help to let him know that the drugs may merely delay his response, and that, with prolonged stimulation, he may achieve erection and orgasm despite his slowed reaction time.

If that doesn't work, switching medications may relieve the problem. Anticholinergics such as mecamylamine (Inversine), adrenergic inhibitors such as guanethidine sulfate (Ismelin) and reserpine (Serpasil), and diuretics like spironolactone (Aldactone) have all been known to affect sexual response; but this reaction is unpredictable and highly individual. A patient who has problems with one of them may well be quite unaffected by another.

* *Can women be sexually impaired by antihypertensives?*

It's well-known that antihypertensive drugs can affect male sexual arousal. Can these drugs also impair female response? If so, how? What can be done about it?

For women, antihypertensives have been implicated in decreased vaginal lubrication and inability to reach orgasm. Some women on antihypertensives also experience a decrease in libido; others retain a strong desire for intercourse but are frustrated by their physiological incapacity to be aroused.

Methyldopa is one antihypertensive whose diminishment of female libido has been well documented. Guanethidine sulfate (Ismelin) causes "dry sex" (failure to ejaculate) in men and is thought to have a comparable effect on female lubrication as well.

The problem can often be relieved by modifying the dosage or switching from one type of antihypertensive to another. Often the difficulty does not arise from the drug alone, but from the drug in combination with such other factors as fatigue, emotional stress, marital discord, alcohol consumption, and concurrent illnesses and medications. If these contributing causes are reduced, your patient's sexual functioning may be restored even if she remains on her antihypertensive.

* Minimizing sex-related pain for arthritics

I am working with a group of chronic arthritics. What advice can I give them about avoiding joint and back pains during intercourse?

Suggest that they plan their intercourse for the time of day when pain is usually least severe. They can prepare by taking analgesic and anti-inflammatory medications. They also can take a warm bath or shower and apply hot packs to afflicted areas. Loosening-up exercises may also help.

Encourage your patients to experiment with a variety of positions to discover which are the most comfortable. Their greatest problems are likely to be keeping weight off the hip and spine and accommodating to a woman's hip contractures. The female superior position usually puts the least amount of strain on an arthritic woman. Your patients also may enjoy positions that permit vaginal entry from the rear or allow them to lie on their sides.

Counseling may prove helpful, too. A sex partner may interpret an arthritic's expression of pain as rejection or might withdraw sexually out of fear of causing injury. Caution against such overreaction. Actually, sex can have an analgesic effect that sometimes lasts for hours.

Persistent sexual dysfunction arising from a hip disability can be an indication for a prosthetic hip replacement. However, prosthetic dislocation during intercourse has been reported. So, if any of your patients have such prostheses, caution them against coital movements that can produce forceful or extreme motions of the hip.

* What to advise arthritics about vibrators

A 73-year-old woman with severe rheumatoid arthritis has asked me about masturbating with a vibrator. What counseling can I offer her?

You can start off by congratulating her on her awareness that sexual satisfaction may be attainable regardless of age or physical infirmity.

If she has a weak or painful grip, she'll probably find a tube-shaped vibrator most comfortable to hold. You might encourage her to experiment freely with it. She's most likely to reach orgasm by applying the vibrator to the clitoral area. For such external use, to cushion vibrations, she may wish to place a clean handkerchief between the machine and the region being stimulated. For internal use, to avoid irritation, it's important to lubricate the surface of the device with K-Y or other water-soluble jelly (petrolatum can interfere with natural vaginal lubrication). She may find her tissues are thin and easily broken. If the cause is atrophic vaginitis, the condition generally can be remedied by estrogen cream (dienestrol or Premarin). However, if the atrophy results from systemic steroids she's taking for arthritis, we'd advise her to use the vibrator sparingly and gently, if at all.

* *Sex in paraplegia*

A newly paraplegic patient wants to know if she'll still be able to experience orgasm and conceive and deliver normally. What can I tell her?

She's probably heard, correctly, that a spinal cord injury generally impairs not only genital sensations but also the pelvic vasocongestion that is associated with arousal and leads to orgasm.

Even so, you can inform her that many paraplegic women do have orgasms. In some cases, they apparently are purely subjective, involving no physical reactions. But in other women, physiological changes associated with orgasm actually occur—not in the genitalia but in other parts of the body that have become erotic zones.

You might tell your patient about a woman we'll call Marilyn, who was seen at the Masters and Johnson Institute's physiology laboratory. Before being cord-injured in a car accident, Marilyn derived little erotic pleasure from stimulation of her breasts. Six months after her injury, however, breast stimulation was producing orgasms complete with many of the usual cardiopulmonary responses to sexual excitation. Furthermore, the Institute reports, the lips of her mouth underwent many of the changes that usually occur in the genital labia: They became engorged to twice their normal size and, at the moment of orgasm, pulsated in waves—with the swelling then dissipating rapidly.

If your patient's reproductive system is undamaged, you can assure her that she'll probably be able to conceive and deliver. She may experience amenorrhea and menstrual irregularity at first, but these rarely

persist beyond a year after the accident. In general, fertility is otherwise unimpaired.

Chances are she'll be able to carry a fetus through a normal term and deliver it vaginally. Still, paraplegics do have high-risk pregnancies, with an increased incidence of cesarean births. Urinary tract infections are a common complication, as most paraplegic women have neurogenic bladders and are at greater risk of ureteral reflux and chronic pyelonephritis.

As the due date approaches, careful monitoring becomes necessary; both labor and fetal monitoring are indicated. There's an increased likelihood of premature labor. Moreover, the paraplegic woman may not feel the contractions, so delivery may be abrupt. Since she's unable to give voluntary assistance in bearing down, Lamaze or other natural childbirth techniques are not appropriate. There's no obstacle whatever to breast-feeding.

Remind your patient that she'll continue to need a contraceptive. Many paraplegic women prefer the IUD; if that's your patient's choice, she'll need periodic gynecological checkups because there's a small risk that the device might perforate her uterus without her feeling it.

A nearly risk-free alternative is foam plus a condom. A diaphragm is too difficult to insert, and the Pill is contraindicated because paraplegics have a predisposition to thrombophlebitis. After your patient no longer wishes to have children, she and her partner might consider tubal ligation or a vasectomy.

* *Impotence from psoriasis*

One of our psoriasis patients suffers from impotence. Is there an association?

There can be. While the inflammatory condition itself has no effect on erection, the skin's appearance may impair the patient's body image and cause imagined or genuine rejection by his partner. Topical medications used for psoriasis, such as coal tar and anthralin (Anthra-Derm), can also be unsightly. Methotrexate, given for severe disabling psoriasis, may cause impotence as a side effect.

A joint counseling session may help a couple come to terms with the esthetic problems posed by the condition. We'd encourage them to explore their reactions to the patient's appearance. We'd also distinguish between the skin and the person, emphasizing the patient's best qualities and his continuing need for love and sexual gratification.

You might suggest that the patient cover his lesions during intercourse. If they're too extensive for bandaging, he might cover them with garments. These can be as simple as a T-shirt or pajamas or more sexually provocative. We know one couple who arranged picnics in secluded areas, regarding it as a "turn-on" to make love outdoors wearing clothing; a female psoriasis patient engaged in sexual activity wearing a sexy leotard with the crotch and other areas cut out. Scheduling coitus before the application of offending topical preparations may also help.

When the impotence is caused by a drug—or if the partner remains resistant to coitus—it's important to inform patients of ways to achieve sexual pleasure without penile-vaginal intromission.

* Risks in intercourse with inguinal hernia

Is there any danger if a male patient with an inguinal hernia engages in sexual intercourse?

The exertion of intercourse could force the bowel into the scrotum, causing pain and possible strangulation of the intestine. Ideally, the hernia should be surgically repaired as soon as possible. However, if your patient refuses surgery, you can suggest that he wear a truss during intercourse. He also can reduce exertion if he forgoes the male superior position in favor of lying on his side or having his partner on top.

* Parkinson's disease: Its sexual effects

One of my clients has Parkinson's disease. What can I say to him about his sexual prognosis?

Most victims of this degenerative neurologic disease suffer from sexual impairment. Symptoms of the disease—arm and leg tremor, muscular rigidity, slowness of movement—make intercourse difficult. Impotence is common, usually a result of advanced organic involvement.

Psychological factors can contribute to your parkinsonism patients' sexual dysfunction. They may be embarrassed by their stooped posture, weak voice, and excessive salivation. Their stiff facial musculature can make them seem dull and slow to respond. They and their loved ones thus tend to withdraw from each other, further decreasing sexual activity. Some patients develop a reactive depression, with reduced libido.

Reassuring couples that a gratifying sexual relationship is possible, despite neuromuscular symptoms, may help; counsel them, too, on the need to take time and have patience. Remind your patient's family, as well, that there's a warm, interested human being behind the glassy parkinsonian mask.

Levodopa therapy is likely to improve your patient's sexual functioning. With improved motor control, there's often increased alertness and a mild euphoria. The glow of well-being tends to heat up sexual activity, giving levodopa the unfounded reputation of being an aphrodisiac.

The drug may also affect your patient's sexual functioning through hormonal changes. Semen may become more copious and viscous. In a postmenopausal woman, the drug may cause increased vaginal secretions (along with uterine bleeding).

* *Contraceptives in sickle cell disease*

What contraceptive method do you advise for women with sickle cell disease?

The safest method for such women is a diaphragm plus spermicidal jelly or cream. For maximum protection, you might teach the patient how to calculate her probable day of ovulation and recommend that her partner use a condom during the three days before and three days after.

Another technique that also affords satisfactory protection is the use of contraceptive foam *plus* a condom. These barrier methods are preferable to oral contraceptives, which can add to the risk of thromboembolic disorders already present in sickle cell disease. IUDs are also contraindicated because the increased risk of hemorrhage and infection can pose a severe hazard to sickle cell patients.

See: Foster HW. Contraceptives in sickle cell disease. *South Med J* 74:543, 1981.

* *What to advise when asthma interferes with sex*

What can be done for a patient whose asthma interferes with sexual intercourse?

He might ward off asthma attacks if he takes an antiallergic prophylactic agent such as cromolyn sodium (Intal) about 30 minutes before engaging in sexual activity. Using a bronchodilator may also increase his ability to function; if an inhalant has been prescribed, assure him that it's perfectly acceptable to use it during lovemaking, if needed. Asthma is often accompanied by anxiety or depression; an appropriate tranquilizer may also improve sexual functioning.

Your patient may benefit from counseling if personality traits contribute to his sex-related attacks. The expectation that his sex partner will know what satisfies him without being told, for example, can result in anger, frustration, and feelings of sexual inadequacy—any of which can trigger an attack. Many asthmatics are task-oriented and develop symptoms because of anxiety about sexual performance.

In addition, suggest that your patient check the bed for allergens. We know one asthmatic who began to wheeze every time he went to bed with his girlfriend. He thought he was afraid of sex, when actually he was sensitive to the down in her quilt.

* *Advising lung patients on resuming sex*

I work in a pulmonary unit. Many of my patients with emphysema, chronic bronchitis, and other chronic lung diseases complain that their shortness of breath keeps them from having intercourse. What can you recommend for their sexual rehabilitation?

To start with, you can reassure your patients that, with sensible preparations, they'll probably be able to tolerate coitus at the frequency they were used to before the onset of their illness. Chronic lung patients are typically anxious that they'll suffocate from the exertion of intercourse and thus may avoid even realistic levels of activity.

A man who is resuming sexual activity after a long period of abstinence is likely to be fearful about his performance. To help him reassure himself of his continued capacity, you might suggest that he engage in low-stress activity the first time or two. This can include cuddling, touching, oral-genital sex, mutual masturbation, or any other source of pleasure that's acceptable to him and his partner.

For regular resumption of intercourse, you might remind patients that lovemaking need not take place at night. It should occur when both partners are feeling freshest, perhaps in the morning or midafternoon. You can suggest that intercourse take place within an hour after taking medications to relieve shortness of breath. Just before coitus, it may help to use a bronchodilator aerosol or inhalator. A patient using oxygen might increase his usual amount by an extra liter per minute, unless his physician says otherwise.

You also might recommend that patients use positions that require the least amount of effort. For men, the female superior position is an energy saver; it also makes it easier for women to achieve orgasm because they have more control over their own stimulation. The lateral position, in which the partners lie on their sides, is suitable for both men and women. A waterbed can be a big help, by creating motion with minimal effort.

In any counseling you do, we'd suggest that you include the sex partner. Point out that resumption of a sex life will greatly enhance the quality of life for the patient, and encourage both partners to express their concerns. Patients with chronic bronchitis or bronchiectasis often have an unpleasant odor to their breath and, as a result, may push away their partners rather than risk rejection. This is the sort of fear that is best talked out in a candid joint session.

See: Davis K. Sexual counseling for the patient with chronic lung disease. *Sex Med Today* 5:10, March 1981.

* *Dealing with a cancer patient who avoids sex*

One of our male cancer patients, who has been hospitalized for several weeks, is avoiding intercourse with his wife during his weekend passes. He argues that sexual pleasure in the face of his death is unnecessary. His wife, however, sees sex at this time as more important than ever. She's brought me the problem. How do I handle it?

Almost certainly you need to bring them both in for an open discussion. We'd suggest you start off by asking what effect they think cancer has on a person's sexuality—and then raise their level of information. He may believe he can give her cancer of the vagina. She may not realize that radiation and medication can decrease his sexual desire.

A good next step is to help her express her need to be close to him. With your assistance, she can make it clear that she wants to feel intimate with him and needs a release for her sexual tension. She can also be explicit about feeling rejected—she may believe his shying away from her is a form of deathbed truth ("So this is how he really feels about me!").

He, in turn, needs a chance to express his feelings about his illness and his sexuality. Surgical mutilation may have made him ashamed of his body. He may be displacing onto his wife his anger over dying.

Simply coping with his physical problems may leave him with little energy for sex. He may suffer from the "I'm already dead" syndrome. One physically capable cancer patient actually told us, "Corpses don't have intercourse."

You can focus on what he still has to give and can take, rather than on what he's losing. Even if he can't get an erection, he nonetheless can be a warm, caring sex partner. Stress that his wife needs him emotionally and that there are many ways he can gratify her sexually. If these techniques don't work, professional counseling may prove helpful.

* *Sexual advice for ostomates*

As an enterostomal therapist, I'm often asked how ostomates might best ready themselves for sexual activity. Any suggestions?

To enhance comfort and ensure cleanliness, you might recommend that an ostomate take a warm, relaxing bath or shower before engaging in sexual activity. It's important to empty the pouch and to protect the bed in case there's an accident. If there's bladder involvement, it's a good idea to catheterize. Men can fold the catheter back alongside the penis and then apply a condom; women can move the catheter out of the way and tape it to the thigh or abdomen.

To encourage sexual rehabilitation, you might stress techniques to help increase enjoyment of sex, such as eliminating time constraints and setting the mood with music, lighting, and wine. The partners could make use of sexually stimulating materials. Women might wear crotchless panties that are not only erotic but also provide a covering for the stoma.

* *Precautions for tracheostomy patients*

What precautions should I advise that a tracheostomy patient take during sexual activity?

During close hugging, the patency of the stoma may be disturbed. Most patients quickly learn to avoid those positions that make it difficult to breathe easily.

You might give your patient a clear understanding of what a trach is—mainly to show that very few special precautions are necessary. Some trach patients worry about oral sex because they're afraid that they'll choke. You need merely depict for them the relationship between the trachea and the esophagus.

* *Can sexual activity trigger a seizure?*

A young woman with petit mal epilepsy has been advised that any type of excitement can trigger a seizure and that she should avoid all emotional extremes. She has never engaged in sexual activity, and now fears that sexual excitement and orgasm will bring on a seizure. How likely is this to occur? What do you advise?

You can reassure this young woman that it's extremely rare for sexual activity to precipitate seizures and that the sexual functioning of most epileptics is unaffected by their disorder.

She can conclusively gauge her own reaction if she brings herself to orgasm. Since she evidently has never masturbated, you may need to reassure her that it's a perfectly valid form of sexual expression. We'd suggest that she explore her sexual responses after a shower, when she's relaxed and feeling good about her body—and in bed, so that if a seizure does occur she won't be injured.

This young woman, however, may be using her expressed fears as an excuse for avoiding undesired sexual activity. Hyposexuality—a reduction in libido—appears to be the most widespread sexual effect of epilepsy. It may be a feature of the disorder. It also may result from feelings—common among patients with epilepsy—of inferiority, social stigmatization, and anxiety and helplessness over their condition.

The reduction in seizure frequency that effective therapy provides may, in itself, increase sexual drive. On the other hand, the sedative side effects of such anticonvulsants as phenytoin (Dilantin) and phenobarbital may lower libido and interfere with the normal reflexes of sexual response. Phenytoin also may cause excessive hair growth and overgrowth of gum tissue, which can lead to feelings of unattractiveness. The dosage of these drugs needs to be carefully titrated by a physician, with sexual and other side effects in mind.

* Female catheterization and intercourse

A female patient of mine will soon be discharged with an indwelling Foley catheter. What sex-related counseling can I offer her?

First, you can assure her that this condition need not rule out intercourse. After disconnecting the Foley from the bag, she can clamp the catheter end and tape it to her leg or abdomen. To avoid bladder discomfort, she might refrain from taking fluids for an hour or so before making love. She and her sex partner may be aware of the catheter at first, but they're likely to soon get used to it.

CHAPTER 4

*

Surgery-related Problems

*

THE PATIENT recovering from almost any type of surgery is likely to be in a dependent position for a long period. Family relationships are often disrupted. There may be financial anxieties. The patient may feel depressed, weak, helpless, and in pain. Some surgical patients feel diminished by the loss of a bodily part. Some feel violated and angry. These emotional reactions to the surgery can interfere with sexual functioning long after the patient has recovered physically.

If the surgery involves the genitals or a female's breasts, the patient's emotional reaction is likely to be intensified. Patients with such surgery almost invariably worry about how it will affect their sex lives.

You might anticipate your patient's concerns by discussing—before the operation as well as afterward—what the sexual effects of the surgery might be. Suggest alternative means of sexual gratification until the patient is ready to resume intercourse. If the underlying condition permanently impairs penile-vaginal intercourse, discuss the wide range of sexual options still available to your patient.

* Sexual advice for mastectomy patients

How does mastectomy affect sexuality? What sort of sex counseling do you recommend?

This is an extremely important question. As a nurse you may be in the best position to relieve one of the great deficiencies of breast cancer care.

Most patients experience breast amputation as a devastating loss. It is almost inevitably equated with a loss of femininity and sexual attractiveness. Yet the impact of mastectomy on a woman's sexual life is rarely addressed. In a Masters and Johnson Institute study, only four of 60 women reported discussing, before surgery, how it might affect their sexuality. Many of the women wanted such counseling, but assumed that it was inappropriate, since no health professionals had brought up the topic.

Many mastectomy patients report that the surgery has a negative effect on their sex lives. In the Masters and Johnson study, frequency of intercourse generally decreased. More women reported never or rarely having coital orgasm. Women who frequently initiated intercourse before surgery rarely did so afterward. The frequency of breast stimulation as a part of sexual activity also declined.

Give your mastectomy patients an opportunity to discuss their anxieties. Typically, a woman's greatest concern is fear of rejection by her husband or other sex partner. She may also fear that person's pity, which implies that she has indeed been diminished.

If possible, involve the partner in discussions about sexual problems. To a great extent, of course, a couple's sexual adjustment after mastectomy depends on the relationship they shared before the operation. But sexual problems may beset even the most loving couple. One common scenario: A postmastectomy patient sees herself as mutilated and repulsive. She thus withdraws from sexual contact. Her partner, feeling rejected, eventually stops approaching her, helping to perpetuate a cycle of misunderstanding. If you help your patients anticipate such reactions, they're likely to deal better with this and related problems. Encourage the couple to speak freely to each other about sex-related concerns.

It's usually a good idea to involve the woman's partner in some of her physical care while she's in the hospital. Massaging her arm, changing her dressing, and other tender, nonsexual physical contact is a good bridge to sexual relations.

Also recommend that your patient join Reach to Recovery, the self-help group for mastectomy patients that's affiliated with the American Cancer Society. We've found this and other such organizations to provide candid, practical advice about sexual problems, prostheses, and related matters.

* *How to counsel after cystectomy?*

What's the sexual prognosis for a man who's undergone a radical cystectomy because of carcinoma of the bladder?

After a radical cystectomy, a man is unable to have an erection because the peripheral branches of the pelvic nerves are interrupted. And he can no longer ejaculate because the surgery entails removal of the prostate and seminal vesicles. With manual or oral stimulation of the flaccid penis, however, he can still experience an orgasm. His testes remain active with sperm being resorbed; so he experiences no feminization.

Such a patient is usually an excellent candidate for surgical implantation of a penile prosthesis. He's likely to be suited to either of the two types: the semirigid silicone rubber prosthesis, which results in a permanent erection; or the inflatable device, which allows him to control the presence or absence of an erection.

Even without a penile prosthesis, the patient needs to be assured that he can enjoy lovemaking and can provide his partner with physical and emotional gratification. The services of an enterostomal therapist—and membership in an ostomy club—can be invaluable in his rehabilitation. Because he has an abdominal urinary stoma and must wear a urinary appliance, he's almost bound to be embarrassed about lovemaking at first. But most men can learn to overcome this.

* *Loss of desire after oophorectomy*

My mother underwent a total hysterectomy and bilateral oophorectomy. Now she says she lacks sexual desire and is unresponsive to intercourse, much to her and my father's frustration. Is there a remedy?

Your mother may have atrophic vaginitis, a postmenopausal degeneration of the vaginal epithelium that may result from oophorectomy. Estrogen cream (dienestrol or Premarin) usually reduces the discomfort and bleeding, thereby promoting sexual arousal and enjoyment of intercourse. We've also seen small amounts of testosterone, given for a short period, improve some women's sense of well-being, which in turn raises their libido.

Your mother needs a gynecological exam, followed by joint counseling with your father if the sexual problem needs further clarification.

* *Prostate resection and sterility*

What should I tell patients to expect sexually after transurethral resection (TUR) of the prostate? Does it cause sterility? Impotence?

For all practical purposes, your patient is likely to be sterile, yet remain potent, after TUR. He'll continue to produce sperm cells and semen as before. But in eight out of 10 cases, ejaculation is retrograde: propelled not forward through the penis but backward into the bladder. That's because the resection often damages the sphincterlike mechanism that ordinarily closes off the bladder during ejaculation. The ejaculate then takes the path of less resistance.

There's nevertheless no organic reason for your patient to be *impotent* after TUR. The procedure interferes with neither the nerve fibers nor the blood flow to the penis. Some TUR patients do suffer psychogenic impotence, but this may be prevented by prompt, but gradual, resumption of sexual activity.

You can reassure your patient that he'll continue to have orgasms. But if he doesn't ejaculate through his penis, he'll lose the pleasant sensation of the semen passing through the urethra.

* Sex after penectomy

A 58-year-old man with penile cancer has had a subtotal penectomy in which 85 percent of his penis was removed. His lymph nodes, prostate, and testicles were left intact. What sexual options are available to him? What sexual responses is he capable of?

Your patient can still experience orgasm, including ejaculation. The penile stump may be capable of erection. Although the glans and frenulum are gone, the bulb of the penis—at the base—can provide highly pleasurable sensations.

With or without erection, your patient may enjoy vaginal intromission. And remind him that most nerve endings in the vagina are situated around the opening, so he may give just as much enjoyment to his partner as he did preoperatively.

He may especially benefit from your pointing out that penile-vaginal contact is only one sexual option. Determine what other forms of sexual activity he has enjoyed, and support him in resuming those.

* Sexual problems after a hysterectomy

How can I help a patient who finds herself unable to have an orgasm since her hysterectomy?

You'd probably be performing a great service if you talked to both the patient and her sex partner. Hysterectomy often makes women feel neutered or makes them suspect that their partners regard them that way. Indeed, your patient's partner *may* be treating her in subtly different ways as a result of her surgery.

Assure both partners that hysterectomy does not physiologically interfere with a woman's ability to enjoy sex. It may be helpful to show, with diagrams, that it's the uterus that has been removed and that the vagina and clitoris are intact.

Clear up any other mistaken notions they may have as well. If the surgery was made necessary by uterine cancer, the partner may feel that he can somehow be contaminated. Explain that hysterectomy alone does *not* cause premature menopause and that, even if the ovaries were also removed, menopausal symptoms can be controlled with estrogens. You can also dispel any myths surrounding hysterectomy that the couple may have picked up, including the mistaken beliefs that it makes a woman hairy, wrinkled, or fat, shrinks her breasts, or causes her to develop a psychosis. You might mention, too, that, after a hysterectomy, freedom from fear of unwanted pregnancy makes many women enjoy sex more than ever.

* *Counseling for husband after hysterectomy*

My husband and I had an excellent sex life until I had a hysterectomy eight years ago. Since then, though he's only in his 50s, my husband claims he is unable to have erections. He says this is due to aging. I've disproved this physiological cause by waiting until he falls into a deep sleep and then manually exciting him. When I tell him he's had erections from such stimulation, he accuses me of lying.

I feel his problem is that he can't cope with my hysterectomy. Somehow, he got the idea that a woman's sexual passion dies with removal of her reproductive organs. I've told him this, but it does no good. How can I change his frame of mind so we can resume our wonderful sexual relations?

While we sympathize with your pain, we doubt that you can resolve the problem without professional assistance. Your husband's unlikely to be convinced by you, and your efforts to act as a therapist could compound complex emotional and attitudinal factors that may be contributing to his impotence. In addition, he may have a circulatory impairment that permits nocturnal erections but not active intercourse.

We'd suggest you both consult a qualified sex therapy team, for a medical workup as well as counseling. You might ask a local medical society or medical school for a referral or query the American Association of Sex Educators, Counselors, and Therapists, 11 Dupont Circle, N.W., Washington, D.C. 20036. The field is overrun with unqualified people, so you'd best seek out reliable recommendations.

* *When to resume sex after abdominal surgery*

I believe that most patients who've undergone bowel resections, appendectomies, and other types of abdominal surgery are interested in when they can return to presurgical sexual activity, whether or not they broach the subject. How should I initiate the discussion? What guidelines can I give them?

You're probably correct in your belief, even though the patients' sexual concerns are rarely expressed by them or dealt with by the staff. A good time to bring up the subject is during your review of discharge instructions, perhaps with a statement like, "Many patients who've had your type of surgery wonder when they can resume sexual activity."

In general (check with the surgeon), the patient can resume intercourse when it's safe to lift 10 pounds or more; this is usually three or four weeks postop, but can be as little as a week, depending on the kind of surgery. At first, a lateral or a recumbent coital position may be most comfortable because it keeps weight off the wound. It's also important to point out that noncoital forms of sexual activity can generally be resumed as soon as the patient feels like it; indeed, if such activities were practiced before surgery, they're to be encouraged.

See: Robusto N. Advising patients on sex after surgery. *AORN J* 32:55, 1980.

CHAPTER 5

*

Genitourinary Problems in Males

*

GENITOURINARY INJURIES, malformations, and infections are commonly associated with changes in sexual functioning or behavior. Your urology patients may suffer from psychogenic sexual disorders, a result of attention being drawn to the sexual organs.

You might take particular care that your patient understands the meaning of the clinical terms you use. A man who is experiencing retrograde ejaculation, for example, should understand that he'll be infertile because his semen is being propelled backward into the urinary bladder. Make sure he knows what the word infertile means and doesn't confuse it with impotent.

* *Pain on ejaculation*

Because my husband finds it painful to ejaculate, he rarely experiences an orgasm when we have intercourse. He suffers no pain when he urinates or at any other time. What causes this condition? How might it be remedied?

Your husband may have a subclinical inflammation of the urethra that causes pain only on ejaculation because of the viscosity of semen. Inflammation may result from an infection or from food allergy or overindulgence in coffee and spicy foods. He might cut out such foods for a week or so. If he still experiences pain, we'd suggest he consult his physician for possible urethritis or prostatitis. Ejaculatory pain also can arise from phenothiazine antipsychotic drugs such as trifuoperazine

(Stelazine) and chlorpromazine (Thorazine) and from psychogenic causes.

* *Causes of penile pain*

A 54-year-old patient complains that his penis hurts during intercourse, causing him to lose his erection. What could be the cause?

Most cases of male dyspareunia we've seen involve insufficient vaginal lubrication, which can cause the uncircumcised male's foreskin to be painfully pulled back and possibly torn or bruised. The best remedy is to improve technique so that the woman is adequately stimulated before intromission. You also might check for balanitis (inflammation of the penis), phimosis (tightness of the foreskin), and paraphimosis (retraction of phimotic foreskin, resulting in swelling of the glans), any of which could cause penile pain that would discourage an erection. We'd also rule out Peyronie's disease, varicosities of the dorsal vein, and thrombosis of the corpora cavernosa—diagnoses that would most reliably be made by a urologist.

* *An overlooked culprit in loss of erection*

My husband constantly loses his erection during intercourse. Our family doctor attributes this to tension, even though we're happily married and under no unusual stress. Sessions with a psychiatrist have led nowhere. Can you suggest the cause?

Your husband may have pelvic steal syndrome, a vascular insufficiency of the penis that usually results from atherosclerosis or trauma. Normally, a patient with the syndrome has enough penile blood supply to achieve a firm erection and to masturbate to orgasm or to penetrate the vagina. But when he moves vigorously, as in active coitus, blood shunts from the penile arterioles to the muscles in his buttocks, legs, and back, causing his penis to become flaccid.

This form of organic impotence is often misdiagnosed as psychogenic because intracoital loss of erection commonly suggests emotional stress. Moreover, the patient has nocturnal erections, which usually leads diagnosticians to mistakenly rule out an organic cause.

The condition is often seen in middle-aged men who have no other cardiovascular symptoms. It also may show up in young men whose physical development is apparently normal but who are unable to complete intercourse. Typically, they've suffered a long-forgotten crush injury or pelvic fracture.

We'd suggest your husband see a urologist for a workup. He'll need a check of his penile blood pressure before and after deep-knee bends, jogging in place, or other exercise. A reduction in penile blood flow from exertion would tend to confirm the syndrome. Arteriography may enable a conclusive diagnosis and lead to vascular repair or a penile prosthesis.

* *Embarrassment from a permanent prosthetic erection*

A patient with a semirigid penile implant has a permanent erection that's a constant source of embarrassment to him and his nurses. How do you advise that we deal with it?

Pretty much as you'd treat any other prosthesis. To deal objectively with the erection, it may help to visualize the twin silicone rods implanted in the corpora cavernosa. Body parts often look different when modified by an appliance. With this type of implant, if no vasocongestion is present, the erection is thinner than one that's turgid from vascular engorgement, and the glans is not enlarged.

You and your colleagues might also become more comfortable with the situation if you reflect on the causes of intractable impotence and the problems erectile dysfunction can create for the patient and his sex partner. Recognizing the value of the implant is likely to help nurses view it more objectively, and such acceptance generally eases the patient's embarrassment.

You also might exchange practical ideas for caring for prosthetic erections. The implants are designed to be flexible, so your patient may be more at ease if he wears jockey shorts. In prepping him or giving him perineal care, you can drape a towel over the penis. If the organ has to be placed to one side, he may prefer holding it there himself.

* *Priapism: Cause and treatment*

Can priapism be caused by prolonged intercourse? Are ice packs an effective treatment?

The onset of priapism—a persistent, abnormal erection of the penis—is often associated with vigorous and prolonged intercourse. But it's likely that the intercourse merely precipitates the condition, rather than causes it. Indeed, the pathologically sustained erection may be what makes the prolonged intercourse possible.

Patients with idiopathic priapism—in which there's no identified cause—often have had transient episodes following intense sexual stimulation. In such cases, a cycle of reflex vascular spasm and edema is thought to obstruct drainage from the erectile tissues.

Most causes of priapism have nothing to do with sexual arousal. Sickle cell anemia, chronic myelogenous leukemia, and polycythemia are among the most common underlying conditions; less frequently, venous obstruction resulting from spinal cord injury or tumors may be the cause. The pathology may also be an effect of phimosis, urethral polyps, urethral calculi, or prostatitis.

Occasionally, priapism may be the result of penile trauma: Hematoma and edema may reduce venous outflow or increase arterial inflow to the corpora cavernosa, causing a persistent erection. Certain drugs—thioridazine (Mellaril), heparin, testosterone, and hydralazine (Apresoline)—have occasionally been reported to bring on the condition.

Whatever the cause, consider priapism an emergency: It can result in damage to the erectile tissue, and sexual function is rarely recovered unless treatment is prompt and effective. Ice packs are among the many remedies, but are rarely adequate alone. The corpora are likely to contain thick venous blood the consistency of motor oil, which may need to be evacuated and irrigated through large-bore (12- or 16-gauge) needles.

Neurologic priapism may be relieved by continuous caudal or spinal anesthesia. A saphenous vein shunt may aid in detumescence by diverting blood from the erectile tissue. The insoluble fibrin may be removed by means of a proteolytic enzyme given intravenously. For priapism caused by trauma, there's usually a need for immediate surgery, with drainage of fluid or blood.

* *Black streaks in semen*

My husband, who is 57, has noticed black and brown streaking in his semen, especially after he's abstained from intercourse for a long time. I want him to see our family doctor, but he feels too embarrassed. Could you offer a suggestion?

We'd recommend he see a urologist—and quickly. The black and brown streaking you describe sounds like hemosiderin, an iron-containing pigment that can derive from accumulated blood. It's sometimes a symptom of bladder cancer and can also indicate inflammation, polyps, and other disorders of the genitourinary system. Occasional hematospermia is rarely a problem, but persistent hematospermia, especially in someone your husband's age, calls for a prompt workup.

* *Blood in semen*

What can cause pink-tinged semen? Does this affect the sperm count? Can it cause chromosomal aberrations? What should be done about it?

This condition is called hematospermia; blood can make the ejaculate appear pink, brownish, or red-flecked. In teenagers and young adults, one of the most frequent causes is hyperemia in the urethral tract. This inflammation, which can occur spontaneously, produces no other symptoms and is self-limiting.

Hematospermia is occasionally a sign of excessive sexual activity, including frequent masturbation; the irritation and capillary rupture that causes it generally resolves after a few days' rest. Hematospermia also may appear in chronic congestive prostatitis; in that case, it would be accompanied by perineal ache, low back pain, pelvic and suprapubic pressure, and frequent painful urination.

Nonspecific urethritis, a sexually transmissible disease caused by the microorganism *Chlamydia trachomatis*, can also cause blood to appear in the seminal fluid; tetracyclines and erythromycin are the most effective treatment options. Yet another possible cause is inflammation or epithelial hyperplasia of the seminal vesicles; the hyperplasia is often treated with 1 mg diethylstilbestrol daily for two to four weeks. Still other possible causes of the condition are urethral polyps and tumors of the seminal vesicles, prostate, vas deferens, and testicles.

There's no chance of hematospermia causing chromosomal aberrations. Since the great majority of cases are benign and self-limiting, we'd suggest being watchful for a week or so. If the condition persists or if other symptoms appear, we'd refer the patient to a urologist for a complete evaluation.

* *What to advise in Peyronie's disease*

What should I tell a man with Peyronie's disease? Does his penis deformity make intercourse impossible?

Reassure him, first of all, that the tender knot on the shaft of his penis is not cancer, a common fear when patients first discover the condition.

You can explain that this hard fibrous tissue is inelastic and thus, as the disease progresses, his erections are likely to become painful. In addition, the erection will curve at the point of fibrosis. This condition is one of the most common causes of male dyspareunia.

Still, your patient has a very good chance of resuming intercourse. About half of the patients with Peyronie's disease recover spontaneously within an average of four years. In the other half, the scarlike region spreads and becomes calcified, making the erect penis bend—usually upward or sideward, but occasionally downward—at an angle of up to 90 degrees. Even so, the pain on erection tends to disappear, and there's often enough flexibility to permit intromission.

Early in the disease, the most widely used medical treatment entails the infiltration of the plaque with steroids, which have an antifibrotic effect. This causes a remission in about 75 percent of cases. If the deformity does become permanent, the plaque can often be removed by surgery, if the fibrosis does not extend too deeply into the penis; otherwise the shaft will have a weak point on erection.

Peyronie's disease typically affects men older than 40. If it doesn't interfere with your patient's sexual functioning, he may accept it as part of aging. Its etiology is uncertain. Some investigators believe that the scar tissue results from an injury or infection possibly due to a virus.

* *How to treat a penis fracture*

What's the physiology of the penile fracture? How is it treated?

Fracture of the penis consists of a tear in any of the three chambers that fill with blood to ıse an erection: the right or left corpus cavernosum or the corpus spongiosum. When the fracture occurs, there may be a crackling sound, with collapse of the erection; intense local pain, penile distortion or discoloration, and the formation of a hematoma, sometimes with urethral injury. Most penile fractures occur during coitus or result from rolling over on an erection or kneading the penis to reduce erection.

Ice packs may be useful first aid to reduce swelling. Good results are reported, for patients who have no urethral injury, with administration of the anti-inflammatory agent oxyphenbutazone (Oxalid, Tandearil), 200 mg q8h for two to three weeks until the hematoma resolves. Diazepam (Valium) is also given as a relaxant, 5 to 10 mg tid or qid.

See: Jallu A, Wani NA, and Rashid PA. Fracture of the penis. *J Urol* 123:285, 1980.

* *What to tell a man with a urethral fistula*

What advice would you give a man who is about to be married and is embarrassed about this condition?

We'd refer him to a urologist or plastic surgeon. Congenital fistulas of the urethra (hypospadias), which cause a male to ejaculate and urinate through an opening on the undersurface of the penis, can generally be repaired surgically without much difficulty. It's best done in infancy, before the age of recall, so the patient isn't troubled with doubts about his sexual adequacy.

You can assure your patient that the condition does not interfere with masculinity. It can, however, lower his chances of conceiving a child if the fistula is so proximal to the scrotum that much of his ejaculate leaks out of the vagina. In rare cases, the penis may be so bent on erection that intromission can be impaired. For one or two months after corrective surgery, operative scarring may cause pain until the scars soften.

* *Adult circumcision*

When one of my patients has an erection, the foreskin can be retracted only about halfway over the glans, making sexual stimulation and manipulation painful. This man has ruled out conventional circumcision as too drastic. Can you recommend an alternative?

Afraid not. Your patient has partial phimosis, one of the principal indications for adult circumcision. Because the foreskin contains a tough fibrous band, efforts to stretch it are painful and rarely effective.

Phimosis can lead to balanitis, chronic irritation, and possibly greater susceptibility to genital herpes and carcinoma of the penis. We'd suggest your patient see a board-certified urologist and discuss ways of making the circumcision as painless as possible, including the use of postop analgesics and tranquilizers to discourage erection.

CHAPTER 6

*

Obstetrical Problems

*

PREGNANCY IS a normal life crisis. Along with its physiological changes, many psychological changes also occur. Among their causes are familial, societal, religious, and cultural conditioning that influence how a woman views pregnancy.

A woman's attitude about her sexuality affects how she responds to the changes that occur throughout the pregnancy year (nine months' gestation, three months' postpartum). If she values her ability to relate to her partner in an intimate manner, she's likely to view her pregnancy as a physical manifestation of such closeness. She'll generally greet the changes in her body with curiosity, excitement, and acceptance.

In marked contrast is the woman who does not value her sexuality and who does not relate well to her partner. For her, the pregnancy may stir up negative feelings about herself and her partner. She's likely to view her body as distorted and ugly. She may complain excessively about the ordinary discomforts of pregnancy. She may doubt her ability to carry the pregnancy to full term.

The husband's attitude toward childbearing and rearing also influences the pregnant couple's adjustment to this normal life crisis. Myths and misconceptions about pregnancy may influence his response and his ability to cope with the changes that pregnancy brings.

As a health professional, you can provide pregnant couples with invaluable information and support during this vulnerable time in their lives. Encourage them to talk about their concerns and about how they are coping with changes in their relationship brought about by the pregnancy. Refer them to childbirth-preparation classes.

It's important for you to impress upon your pregnant patient that she should be tested as soon as possible if there's any possibility that she has a sexually transmitted disease. Let her know that during pregnancy a venereal disease may be harmful not only to her but also to her infant. Make sure she understands that she may have a disease without showing any symptoms.

Sexual intercourse can ordinarily continue throughout a normal pregnancy. But couples should not engage in intercourse after the membranes have ruptured or if the woman has a history of premature labor. Another important caveat: If a pregnant woman experiences vaginal or abdominal pain or bleeding during intercourse or at any other time, caution her to abstain from intercourse until she consults a physician.

When intercourse is proscribed during pregnancy, advise couples to consider this an opportunity to expand their sexual repertoire. Many of the following questions deal in greater detail with sex during pregnancy.

* *Intercourse during pregnancy*

To what extent is intercourse contraindicated during pregnancy?

Vaginal bleeding, ruptured membranes, and a history of premature labor are the major contraindications. Otherwise, in a normal pregnancy, intercourse is in no way harmful to the mother or fetus. Most couples don't abstain for the traditional six weeks before and after delivery and there's no real reason why they should. Following delivery, intercourse can be resumed as soon as the episiotomy heals and it's comfortable, though couples vary widely in their timing on this. Needs and desires differ, and often both parents need help in adjusting to the demands placed on them by the new baby.

In any event, warn your patient that if she and her mate use contraception, it will be needed right off. We know of women becoming pregnant less than a month postpartum.

* *Can sexual activity cause fetal distress?*

I am in my eighth month of pregnancy. Following intercourse, especially when orgasm occurs, my uterus will go into a long painless contraction lasting seven to 10 minutes. Is this harmful to the fetus?

You're describing Braxton Hicks's contractions, a normal part of pregnancy. Usually such contractions occur spontaneously; in many women they're also triggered by sexual activity, which can cause the uterus to go into spasm.

Even the longest such contractions are unlikely to cut off the fetal oxygen supply. If the placenta is intact and the fetus is in good health, the fetus will compensate with an increased heart rate. Penile penetration or even the weight of the sex partner poses no special hazard.

If you're still concerned about the safety of the fetus, consult your obstetrician. He may recommend nonstress tests, which measure the accommodation of the fetal heart. He also may suggest taking a series of estriol levels to determine the well-being of the fetoplacental unit; a decrease indicates that the fetus is compromised. If a fetal heart doesn't make adequate accommodation for contractions, orgasm should be avoided.

* Coital positions for late pregnancy

A woman in late pregnancy complains that her large abdomen interferes with the usual coital position. What positions and/or techniques do you recommend?

Your patient is probably used to the "missionary" position (face-to-face, man on top). This supposedly was the coital position insisted upon by Christian missionaries—and ridiculed by natives who thought it unimaginative.

Suggest that your patient and her partner experiment with any position they find comfortable; this can be a good opportunity for them to break down inhibitions. A pregnant woman often prefers a female superior position (face-to-face, woman on top). It allows her to control the degree of penile penetration and accommodate her enlarged abdomen by sitting higher or raising herself with her arms.

A lateral position (partners on their sides) is another alternative. Suggest that the woman rest on the man's inner thigh and that he place his upper leg between her thighs. This position allows great freedom of movement and makes it relatively easy for the man to accommodate his pelvis to his pregnant partner's abdomen.

Yet another possibility is a rear-entry position, in which the woman lies on her side with her belly supported by the bed. For easier vaginal penetration, her hips may be elevated with a pillow.

During pregnancy, caution couples against sexual activity that may give the woman an air embolism. Her uterus is highly vascular; any sharp rise in air pressure may force a bubble into a blood vessel. Some conservative specialists even recommend that a woman in the last trimester of pregnancy avoid the so-called doggy position—rear entry while the woman supports herself on her knees and her chest or arms. This raising of her pelvis can possibly cause an air pocket to form in her drooping anterior vaginal wall. In theory, vigorous penile thrusting may then pump air into the uterus, causing an embolism. We know of no embolisms actually resulting from this, however, and tend to regard the avoidance of the doggy position as highly precautionary.

* *Yeast infection during pregnancy*

A pregnant patient has a resistant vaginal yeast infection. Is intercourse safe for her? Her husband? The fetus?

Yes, for all concerned. *Candida* poses no hazard to an embryo or fetus and doesn't usually survive in the penis. However, during flare-ups, your patient may prefer nonvaginal forms of sexual activity. Vasocongestion can make the vulvovaginal area more sensitive during pregnancy, and the itching and inflammation of candidiasis can increase discomfort. You can reassure the patient that the condition will probably be easier to clear up after delivery.

* *Postepisiotomy virginity*

Is it true that after having an episiotomy a woman's vagina is once again in a "virgin" state? A multipara tells me her husband swears she's back to her "original fit" each time she has a baby. I used to fear having a baby because of the episiotomy, but now wonder if it might be to my advantage.

While the miracles of modern medicine don't include restoring virginity, your patient's husband is correct in what he senses: To prevent undue laceration during childbirth, a midline episiotomy incises the muscle between the posterior vaginal and anterior rectal walls. During the episiorrhaphy, the surgeon may go beyond the incision and make the introitus smaller than he found it. This can offset the stretching that the vaginal opening undergoes as a result of intercourse.

If you do decide to have a baby, discuss the episiorrhaphy with your doctor. Some obstetricians are loath to give those extra few stitches. Others may make the introitus too tight, a frequent cause of coital pain.

* *A tightened vagina and noisy flatus*

After the birth of my daughter, my obstetrician repaired the episiotomy with "husband knots," an extra few stitches to tighten the vaginal opening. This has made intercourse more pleasurable, but ever since, I've been unable to expel flatus silently. Can you tell me what causes this embarrassing problem and what I can do about it?

Chances are the flatus sounds are unrelated to the reduction of your vaginal opening. More likely, the episiotomy extended to your rectal sphincter. In repairing it, a noise-promoting configuration like a reed or tube may have been formed in the tissue. We suggest you see a proctologist.

* *Timing sex and pregnancy after a cesarean*

How long after a cesarean delivery should a patient avoid pregnancy? When is it safe for her to resume intercourse?

To give the uterus enough time to heal, she should keep from becoming pregnant for at least 12 weeks. She and her partner can usually resume intercourse after four to six weeks—provided her abdominal scar is healed, there's no bleeding or other postpartum discharge, and she's otherwise comfortable.

* *Intercourse and miscarriage*

The current literature says intercourse during pregnancy does not cause miscarriage. Yet the same articles often advise abstaining during the first trimester if there's a history of miscarriage. Isn't this inconsistent?

Obstetrically yes, but psychologically no. Miscarriages generally result from faulty germ cells. It's speculated that fewer than 1 percent of all miscarriages are due to poor implantation, which might possibly be affected by the contractions of the uterus during orgasm.

But too many women believe that sexual activity can "shake loose" an embryo. If a miscarriage results, they are likely to feel guilty about having had orgasms while pregnant. What's more, with each miscarriage, a woman has a higher and higher risk of miscarrying again—and so of feeling even more guilty.

To prevent such guilt, obstetricians often prescribe placebo regimens for women who've had three or more miscarriages. So that a patient can tell herself she's done all she can to prevent yet another one, she's advised to abstain from sex during the first three months of pregnancy—not for the whole month but merely during the days in which she'd ordinarily be having her period.

* *Timing postabortion intercourse*

How soon after an abortion can a patient safely resume intercourse?

Generally she needs to wait until at least 48 hours after the cessation of all bleeding. This usually occurs a week to 10 days after the abortion.

If intercourse is resumed prematurely, bleeding may increase. Moreover, the cervix is still open. During coitus, the penis can act like a plunger, pushing vaginal flora into the uterus and causing pelvic inflammatory disease.

Your patient may actually want to wait a good deal longer than this minimum physiological requirement. After an abortion—be it spontaneous, therapeutic, or elective—many women suffer from grief, guilt, or remorse. Until they resolve such feelings, they're rarely psychologically ready for intercourse. You may do well to recommend qualified postabortion counseling for your patients.

Also, to avoid obstetric complications, advise your patient to wait at least three months before trying to get pregnant again. That's the amount of time needed for the uterus to get back to normal and again be ready for implantation.

* *Pregnancy without intercourse*

A high-school girl is pregnant, although she has an intact hymen and says she's never had intercourse. She has, however, engaged in heavy petting, including mutual masturbation. Am I correct in my suspicion that this could have led to insemination?

Indeed you are. Even though the boy ejaculates extravaginally, any sperm that reaches the girl's vulvar mucosa may lead to fertilization. Such inadvertent insemination may occur through gravity, by way of a finger or other object, or even if the girl's underpants get dampened by the ejaculate. This is important information to pass on to youngsters, who often engage in this form of sexual activity without realizing its risks.

* Pros and cons of circumcision

What should I advise new parents about circumcision?

First of all, you can tell them that the procedure automatically eliminates problems due to the buildup of smegma, the odorous, irritating secretion that accumulates under the foreskin. In the uncircumcised male, daily retraction of the prepuce and washing of the penis is required to remove the smegma. Since this is not always convenient, uncircumcised males are at higher risk of penile inflammations and infections than are circumcised ones. In addition, circumcision may be required later in life—when it's more traumatic than in infancy—if there are recurrent infections of the glans and foreskin or if the foreskin becomes difficult to retract (phimosis) or constricted behind the glans (paraphimosis).

Circumcision is rarely medically necessary and involves a minor risk of infection. There are also rare instances of hemorrhage and surgical mutilation.

You might point out to parents, however, that circumcision is medically necessary if the infant has phimosis or paraphimosis, especially with difficulty in voiding. Conversely, the procedure is contraindicated if there is any displacement of the urethral meatus, since the prepuce may be used later in plastic repair. It is also inadvisable if the infant is in any distress, if there is a family history of hemophilia or another bleeding disorder, or if the mother has been taking anticoagulants, aspirin, or other medication associated with bleeding. Even in Judaism and Islam, which require circumcision, these health considerations justify postponing the ritual.

If a child *is* circumcised, for the first 24 hours afterward, place sterile petrolatum gauze over the area and change it after each voiding. Observe him hourly for bleeding. Position him and his diaper to avoid friction. If the child is discharged before the wound is healed, advise the parents to change his diapers often or to leave him undiapered and to notify the physician if the baby develops a fever greater than 101°F, bright red bleeding, or a rash, swelling, or inflammation.

* Arousal from breast-feeding

A new mother complains of feeling sexually aroused while breast-feeding her baby. What should I tell her?

You can tell her this is an extremely common experience among nursing mothers and that she might simply enjoy it as a reward from nature.

There's an overlap between the nurturing and erotic functions of the breast; both breast-feeding and sexual intercourse stimulate the hormones oxytocin and prolactin, and milk is often ejected during coitus. If your patient's guilt or fear persists, despite your explanation, you might explore whether she has conflicts about her sexuality or her infant.

* Painful intercourse from breast-feeding

Many breast-feeding mothers in my ob/gyn clinic complain of painful intercourse months after delivery. Is there a relationship between nursing and dyspareunia? What advice can I give?

During the postpartum period, there is a relative steroid starvation, causing dryness and thinning of the vaginal mucosa. Breast-feeding can contribute to such a steroid deficiency. To facilitate penetration, you might recommend the use of a water-soluble lubricant or contraceptive jelly. An estrogen vaginal cream (dienestrol or Premarin) may relieve the condition, although some physicians fear that the amount of estrogen absorbed into the breast milk can be harmful to the infant.

Also, we remind couples that caring for a baby generally causes fatigue and emotional tension, which can make it difficult for them to become sexually aroused. Having someone take the baby for a few hours on the weekend can usually help them catch up on sleep and make love while feeling refreshed.

* Effect of sex play on breast milk

In the last trimester of pregnancy and during breast-feeding, can oral stimulation of the breasts during sex play stimulate milk flow? Could this reduce the amount of milk available for the infant?

During the last trimester, the engorgement of the breasts from sexual arousal can cause a leakage of colostrum, the precursor of milk. After delivery, for as long as the mother is lactating, increased blood flow to the breasts during sexual excitement can cause milk to leak. Far from diminishing the amount left for the infant, such practice ordinarily stimulates the breasts to produce more milk, much as if it resulted from the infant's sucking.

CHAPTER 7

*

Gynecologic Problems

*

GYNECOLOGIC PROBLEMS are commonly associated with changes in sexual functioning or behavior. Disorders of the genitals or reproductive system may impair sexuality by affecting body image or self-esteem, by precluding childbearing, or by causing pain or discomfort during sexual activity.

Perhaps the most common gynecological problem is monilial vaginitis, caused by the yeast *Candida albicans*. Be particularly alert for yeast infection in your female patients with diabetes or Addison's disease. It's also more common during pregnancy and in women using oral contraceptives or broad-spectrum antibiotics.

When a patient presents with candidiasis, it may be prudent to screen her for sexually transmitted diseases. The symptoms of yeast in fection—intense pruritus and a thick, cheesy discharge—may mask gonorrhea or syphilis.

A far greater challenge to the health professional is the care of patients with gynecological malignancies. Typically, a woman suffering from gynecologic cancer wants closeness and reassurance from her partner. Encourage such women to talk about sexual concerns. Even when intercourse is impossible, hugging, touching, and sexual contact may continue to be an important part of her life.

To be of most help to patients and their sex partners, discuss with them how cancer and its treatment may affect sexual functioning. Offer counseling regarding resumption of sexual activity. If coitus is precluded, include a discussion of other sexual options. During follow-up care, routinely inquire about sexual problems.

* *Managing stubborn postcoital UTI*

What accounts for urinary tract reinfections following intercourse? Can these flareups be prevented? What's the recommended treatment?

In women, mechanical irritation combined with perineal migration of *Escherichia coli* cause most UTI recurrences related to intercourse. Irritation can be reduced by adequately lubricating the vagina prior to intromission. Cleansing the perineum before coitus may wash away infective organisms.

UTI is often associated with stagnation of residual urine in the bladder, which promotes bacterial growth. It may help for the woman to flush her bladder and urethra after coitus by voiding and then drinking a glass of water to induce mild diuresis.

One effective drug regimen for prophylaxis is trimethoprim-sulfamethoxazole (Bactrim, Septra), half a tablet taken every other day at bedtime. This dosage reportedly can be taken for years with little risk of side effects. However, we rarely find such low-dose, long-term administration necessary and indeed fear that it may promote the development of resistant organisms. Getting rid of UTI recurrences tends to improve the patient's sex life; with the threat of infection gone, a woman is likely to have intercourse more frequently and enjoy it more.

* *How to relieve chronic yeast infection*

What do you recommend for chronic yeast infection? All the medications I take are minimally effective for a few weeks, and then there's a recurrence of the vulvovaginitis and cheesy discharge. Are there long-term effects from the condition? Is sexual intercourse contraindicated?

Recurrent candidiasis (moniliasis) infections require a prolonged, varied attack, because resistant strains of the infecting organism, *Candida albicans*, are sometimes part of the normal flora of the vagina. We get very good results with a 10-day routine that includes intravaginal application of miconazole nitrate (Monistat cream), plus the insertion of gentian violet-impregnated tampons (Genapax) before bedtime and on getting up. In addition, the vulvovaginal area should be painted with gentian violet once a week. We also recommend thrice-weekly douching with yogurt (one tablespoon of active culture in one quart of warm water) for a period of three weeks.

To promote circulation of air, we advise patients to temporarily refrain from wearing underpants and to wear instead crotchless pantyhose or stockings with a garter belt. Similarly, we suggest that they not wear jeans or slacks. In fact, susceptible women should always avoid nylon undergarments and tight pants. They should be especially careful in warm weather and when bodily resistance to infection is lowered, as during periods of illness or emotional stress. Oral contraceptives and broad-spectrum antibiotic therapy also may contribute to the development of candidiasis. Since the infection often occurs in association with diabetes and Addison's disease, it's prudent to rule out those conditions.

We've seen no long-lasting effects after candidiasis is cleared up. If mucosal tenderness doesn't make intercourse uncomfortable, there's no reason not to continue having coitus. *Candida* doesn't seem to affect men, so a sex partner is not at risk. If you're using gentian violet, let your partner know, because it may turn his penis purple. One man called us up at 3 a.m., fearing that his penis was gangrenous and about to fall off.

* Dealing with honeymoon cystitis

What advice can be given to a young newlywed experiencing what seems to be honeymoon cystitis?

Honeymoon cystitis typically results from the woman's not being adequately aroused prior to intromission. Her vaginal dryness leads to irritation, and the inflammation can extend to the urethra. The edematous tissue often becomes infected by retrograde flow, and bacteria may invade the bladder.

This sequence of events can occur at any time. But newly married couples commonly have an increased frequency of intercourse; sometimes they don't really want to, but think they're supposed to. If they take a few days' rest, the condition may go away by itself. A urine culture is needed if the urgency and burning persist or if the symptoms worsen or include hematuria or fever.

The most important preventive is to teach the couple the necessity for adequate stimulation of the female. We'd suggest you counsel both partners conjointly about the male and female sexual response cycles. Point out that the male may sometimes be more easily aroused than his partner and penetrate prematurely, possibly because he fears he'll lose his erection. It may help if you assure him that, by waiting until his wife is ready, he'll not only retain his erection but will find the experience heightened by her pleasure.

Encourage the couple to express explicitly to each other what they find pleasurable—and what they don't care for. You also might tell newlyweds not to expect to feel the earth move every time they make love; young couples are often disappointed when their unrealistic expectations are not met.

* *Allergic reaction to semen*

A woman complains of vaginal burning and vulvar discomfort after having intercourse with her husband. She has had no similar problems from coitus with other men. Can you suggest an explanation?

What you're describing is consistent with an allergy to semen. Allergic seminal vulvovaginitis is usually marked by vaginal burning, stinging, and pain; the vulva may be red, swollen, and urticarial. Symptoms start during coitus or immediately after ejaculation and last from two to 72 hours. In severe cases, the women may need emergency treatment for asthma or anaphylactic shock.

Your patient may be allergic to an active substance in her husband's semen that she hasn't encountered in the semen of other men. However, an allergic woman typically has a reaction to semen in general, since the most frequent antigens are proteins that occur normally in prostatic and seminal fluids.

To confirm the allergy, she can take a specimen of her husband's semen to an allergist for a skin test; a positive reaction will show within 30 minutes. She might be tested with semen from another male to check the specificity of her reaction to her husband.

The patient can avoid the problem by asking her husband to use a condom. As for medication, diphenhydramine (Benadryl) is sometimes effective in preventing vulvovaginal reactions. Attempts at desensitization have not yet proven successful.

* *Vaginitis from designer jeans*

Since buying a pair of $50 designer jeans, a patient has come down with several episodes of coliform vaginitis. Is there a connection?

Very possibly. We've seen pairs of these jeans so tight that the wearer has to put them on while lying down. The resulting perineal sweating promotes the migration to the vagina of any intestinal flora that are contaminating the anal region.

One preventive measure is to wear jeans that are looser around the seat—but that, of course, is just what people want to avoid. So, if your patient insists on wearing her skin-tight jeans, we'd suggest she cleanse her perineal region after each bowel movement. For times when soap and water aren't at hand, as in public rest rooms, she can carry packages of foil-wrapped towelettes.

* *Treatment for clitoral boils*

Are recurrent boils on the clitoris sexually transmitted? What's the best treatment?

The clitoral area is rich in sebaceous glands, which are subject to staph or strep infection, forming a boil (furuncle). The bacteria are resident flora and need not be introduced sexually. However, they're most likely to invade inflamed tissue, which can result from sexual activity.

A single boil is best treated with intermittent moist heat to allow the lesion to point and drain spontaneously. Excision is usually a mistake because it can spread the infection. Multiple boils may be treated with a penicillinase-resistant penicillin such as cloxacillin sodium (Tegopen).

* *Examining a child with vulvovaginitis*

What's the best way to examine a prepubertal girl with vulvovaginitis?

First, before having the child undress, we reduce her apprehension by describing the procedure in detail. We use the words she understands ("You'll lie down with your bottom up so we can see if it's red") and we assure her that the exam won't hurt. To further calm her, we ask her mother to be present during the exam, to hold her hand and otherwise lend support. Because the preadolescent vaginal mucosa is extremely fragile, all entering fingers and objects must be very well lubricated—and warm.

The knee-chest position provides a good view of the vagina and cervix without instrumentation; the vagina is short and usually gapes open if the child lets her abdomen sag and takes a few deep breaths. An ordinary otoscope head, without a speculum, provides adequate magnification and light. To obtain specimens for wet preparations and cultures, we have the child lie supine so she can watch without becoming anxious. Then we gently insert into the vagina a soft plastic eyedropper or saline-moistened cotton applicator.

Since the child is apt to dislike a rectal exam, it's a good idea to leave it for last. In general, a rectal exam is necessary only if there's abdominal pain, vaginal bleeding, or an unusual history. Have the child lie supine with her knees apart and feet together. You can tell her that the exam feels "like going to the bathroom." A bimanual rectal abdominal exam can detect abnormal masses or tenderness.

See: Emans SJ and Goldstein DP. The gynecologic examination of the prepubertal child with vulvovaginitis: Use of the knee-chest position. *Pediatrics* 65:758, 1980.

* What causes pelvic "click"?

My daughter says that during her last pelvic exam she heard a sharp clicking noise in her vagina. She's afraid something broke inside her. Can you suggest an explanation?

Chances are her gynecologist was using a disposable clear plastic speculum whose cogwheel makes that noise when it's opened. Why didn't she ask him directly? If she's intimidated by him, we'd suggest she switch to a doctor with whom she's comfortable.

* Effect of semen on vaginal smears

Would a Pap test or vaginal culture be affected if the patient had sexual intercourse a few hours before and semen were still present? Is douching advisable in such a case?

No on all counts. Semen is sterile, and so wouldn't affect cultures for vaginal infections.

In Pap smears, semen is easily distinguished from the exfoliated cells that are the subject of the cytology. In fact, the patient shouldn't douche for at least three days before the test, because douching would mechanically remove exfoliated cells.

* Little need for hymenectomy

Would a young woman contemplating her first intercourse benefit from a hymenectomy?

Only if her hymen is too thick or fibrous for comfortable intercourse. The introitus should be able to accommodate two fingers, and in the great majority of cases, the patient can self-dilate digitally. Several times a week, preferably while in a warm bath, she should exert pressure along the posterior vaginal wall. If she's been using tampons, the chances are her hymen has already been adequately stretched.

A woman who worries about painful first intercourse may be expressing more general fears about sex or her intended partner. In counseling such a patient, it's a good idea to elicit all the related problems she has on her mind.

When we encounter such fears in a virgin female, we give her a good look at her vulva. Some women believe the hymen is mountainlike in its impassability. So, using a mirror, we point out that her hymen is not the barrier she fears it is. We insert two fingers, to reassure her that penile penetration can take place without pain.

* *Bleeding after intercourse in a teenage girl*

What does it mean when a teenage girl occasionally experiences vaginal bleeding after intercourse?

It means she ought to see a gynecologist. Such bleeding can occur as a result of vaginal infection, cervical erosion, or cervical dysplasia. A tough hymenal ring can also bleed on several occasions after the initial intromission.

A frequent reason for vaginal bleeding among teenagers is irritation and tearing resulting from inadequate lubrication. This is a common problem among girls who aren't ready for intercourse yet feel pressured to engage in it. Such conflicts often obstruct sexual arousal. If pathology is ruled out, you might help your patient sort out her feelings and learn to say "No" when she so prefers.

In addition, your patient's partner may not be providing sufficient sexual stimulation prior to penetration. You could encourage the patient to assert her wishes.

* *Dangers of douching*

Is douching advisable after intercourse or menstruation?

No. In fact it's *in*advisable. The vaginal mucosa cleanses itself. Douches can destroy natural flora if used excessively. Perfumed brands can provoke allergic reactions.

A nurse-patient recently presented with a vaginal infection, marked by red, shiny, edematous, extremely irritated mucosa. She had been douching daily. Then, when she noticed some vaginal odor, she increased her douching to two or three times a day. She now had a clean but angry vagina.

It is, however, good hygiene to wash the external genitalia frequently with soap and water. This does more to decrease odor than does internal cleansing with a douche.

* *Relieving genital varicosities*

Several of my patients suffer discomfort from genital varicosities, either at the end of their pregnancies or at phases of their menstrual cycle. What suggestions for relief might I offer?

To improve circulation, they might take sitz baths at comfortable temperatures for 15 minutes four times a day. They may also try losing weight, keeping off their feet, and taking 15-minute rests with their legs and hips elevated. Some women get relief by applying perineal pressure with two or more sanitary napkins held in place by panties or a belt.

For decreased congestion in the area, we'd advise them to maintain regular bowel habits with proper diet, fluids, and exercise. Discourage straining; if necessary, a stool softener may be recommended by the physician. Also warn them against wearing maternity girdles; constraining the pelvis can aggravate their varicosities.

Genital varicosities are common during pregnancy and usually disappear six to eight weeks after delivery. If chronic genital varicosities become painful or thrombosed, surgical removal of the thrombus and ligation of the vein are usually required.

* *Causes of cervical tenderness*

A patient complains that her cervical area is tender with deep penetration during intercourse. What could account for her discomfort?

She needs a pelvic exam to be certain. The cervix has few nerve endings, so the pain is likely to be referred from other sources.

A rectum full of feces can also cause discomfort with deep penile thrusting. Other possible causes include adhesions, endometriosis, pelvic inflammatory disease, and an inflamed retroverted uterus.

* *Sex after cerclage for incompetent cervix*

What does cerclage for an incompetent cervix entail? How soon after it can a pregnant woman resume sexual intercourse? What are the danger signs she should watch for?

A woman is considered to be suffering from an incompetent cervix when she has had two or more miscarriages due to the spontaneous opening of the cervix within the first trimester. In cerclage, the cervix is sutured early in pregnancy to keep it from opening, and the patient is put on bed rest and limited activity for six to 10 weeks.

Because she must do nothing that might stimulate contractions, we advise against her having intercourse until after delivery. She should also avoid orgasm by other means. Under normal circumstances, sexual activity will not induce premature labor, but, for an incompetent cervix, we regard these precautions to be prudent because the condition poses such high risks.

Warn your patient to be examined immediately if she experiences vaginal bleeding or painful contractions. Also prepare her for the choices that need to be made in regard to the cerclage sutures. For a vaginal delivery, the sutures would be removed to allow the cervix to open. However, recerclage is often difficult because of cervical scar tissue. After having one child, patients frequently elect to have a tubal ligation. Alternatively, especially if the woman wishes to have more children, the sutures may be kept in place, and the delivery is by cesarean section.

* *Causes and cures of hirsutism*

A female patient has thick breast and facial hair. What could account for it? What's the best treatment for this condition?

If the hirsutism appeared abruptly, we'd check what drugs your patient's taking. The antihypertensive minoxidil (Loniten) causes hirsutism in about 80 percent of patients. Other drugs that can cause excess hair growth include androgens, corticosteroids, phenytoin (Dilantin), and diazoxide (Hyperstat, Proglycem).

For hirsutism of unknown etiology, a workup by an endocrinologist may be required; the condition can result from androgenic hormone disorders and from tumors or hyperplasias of the ovaries or adrenal glands.

Most hirsutism is an idiopathic cosmetic problem. As a result of heredity, the woman has body or facial hair that's coarser, darker, or faster-growing than this culture decrees is the esthetic norm for females. For most parts of the body, shaving offers the simplest way to remove hair. You can tell patients that shaving doesn't stimulate hair growth, but does have to be done frequently to avoid a bristly appearance.

Other simple, inexpensive methods include bleaching the hair with hydrogen peroxide or removing it with depilatories (for example, Nair, Neet). Our patients tell us that plucking hair or stripping it with wax is painful and a nuisance.

Electrolysis is the only method for removing unwanted hair permanently. This procedure is often accompanied by needless pain and expense, so we'd advise patients to seek a well-qualified electrologist.

* *Lift for sagging breasts*

Women patients are frequently concerned about their breasts sagging after pregnancy. What causes this to happen? Can it be remedied with surgery? Does wearing a bra help?

The increase in breast size during pregnancy, especially for multigravidas and large-breasted women, can stretch the fragile breast ligaments, giving the breasts a flat, pendulous appearance. Breast sagging may also follow significant weight loss. Some flattening is a normal part of the aging process.

Surgery can relieve sagging breasts by cutting out excess tissue. Within three to five years, however, the sagging usually returns.

Wearing a properly fitting bra can help reduce sagging; bralessness takes its toll in unduly stretched ligaments. You might advise patients to try on each bra they buy to make sure the fit is correct; sizes can vary greatly even within the same brand. A woman should be hardly aware that she is wearing a bra; it shouldn't restrict movement or deep breathing, and there should be no bulge of flesh above the bra or at the underarm. The "strap test" can detect a bra that's too loose: Dropping one strap shouldn't affect support on that side.

* *What to do for inverted nipples*

What can be done for inverted nipples? Are they hereditary? Can plastic surgery correct the condition?

We've never heard of plastic surgery being used to permanently evert a nipple. Nor would we recommend such an operation. Inverted nipples are normal and quite common. They raise cosmetic questions only because of unrealistic fantasies of the female body.

One exception: An everted nipple that suddenly becomes inverted may be a sign of breast cancer and requires evaluation. Otherwise, inverted nipples seem to be hereditary or otherwise inborn; they don't result from tight bras or poor diet, as some people think. They rarely cause serious problems in breast-feeding. Pressure on the areola causes the nipple to protrude so it may be placed in the infant's mouth. Breast shields are often helpful. If these measures don't work, a breast pump may be used.

* *Relief for sensitive nipples*

My nipples are extremely sensitive and hurt if they're touched during sex play, much to my husband's frustration and my displeasure. Can you suggest anything that can help me enjoy nipple stimulation?

You might try rubbing your nipples daily with a towel to help toughen them. During sex play, you can see if the use of oil, saliva, or other lubrication makes fondling your nipples more pleasurable. It's also possible that your husband is touching your nipples too early in your sexual response cycle. If he waits until you're more aroused and then works up to touching your areola by first caressing your entire breast, you may find nipple stimulation enjoyable—especially if you tell him how you'd like it done (fast, slow, light, heavy).

CHAPTER 8

*

Menstruation and Menopause

*

MANY WOMEN greet menstruation and menopause with more than a little ambivalence. Both are rife with myth and misconception.

Without being aware of it, most people have been affected by centuries of adverse religious teaching about menstruation. Leviticus 15:19–30 typifies such teaching. It commands that a woman who has an "issue" of blood shall be put apart for seven days. "And everything that she lieth upon in her separation shall be unclean." Whoever touches her or her bed or other objects shall be "unclean" until evening and must wash himself and his clothes. After seven days have elapsed, and a woman's period is over, she is commanded to bring sacrifices to a priest, who "shall make an atonement for her before the Lord for the issue of her uncleanness." Among Orthodox Jews, intercourse remains forbidden during menstruation.

The effects of this kind of attitude still linger, even among the irreligious. There are also many superstitions about menstruation: A permanent wave will not take on a menstruating woman; her plants will die; her meat will spoil; her bread will fail to rise. Further, menstruation is often presented to young girls in a negative way: it is "the curse," a time when a woman is "unwell."

Some young girls experience this transition to womanhood mainly with pride, wonderment, and anticipation. But others, anxious about their emerging sexuality, may feel shame and disgust.

A woman's experience of menopause may be similarly fraught with ambivalence. She may be influenced by society's negative stereotype of the menopausal woman: hysterical, absurd, on her way to becoming a dried-up old prune. She may fear that she'll lose her interest in sex and her sexual attractiveness.

Further, she may feel deeply the loss of her reproductive capacity. And since menopause often coincides with grown children leaving home, she may also painfully feel the loss of her childrearing functions and perceive herself as useless, inadequate, unfulfilled.

Help your patients see that both menstruation and menopause are normal developmental crises and parts of a woman's continual unfolding as a sexual being. Encourage a menopausal woman to build on other aspects of her personality to develop new interests or build or renew a career.

* *Intercourse during menstruation*

Many of my patients are reluctant to have intercourse during menses. Is it safe?

Yes. You can reassure patients that there's no physiological reason to abstain. Menstrual flow contains an ounce or two of blood, plus cells and tissue fluid from the degenerating layers of the endometrium. Despite widely held fears, it is not "unclean" or in any way harmful to either partner. Nor is it likely that coital thrusting will force menstrual fluid into the fallopian tubes.

Indeed, some couples find intercourse especially enjoyable during menses. The very moist vagina can enhance sensation, and the woman's pelvic vasocongestion may heighten her orgasm. This, in turn, may relieve her menstrual cramps, which are caused by the vasocongestion.

Chances are some of your patients are loath to have intercourse during menses because of their cultural background (it violates Jewish religious law, for instance). If that's the case with a female patient, you may find that she's particularly disturbed by the increase in sexual desire that often occurs at the start of a period. You can reassure her that this is a normal reaction to pelvic vasocongestion, hormonal changes, and lessened fear of pregnancy.

Other couples may be discouraged by the supposed messiness. A diaphragm can contain menstrual discharge. Towels under the couple can protect the bedding. And, because many a man is put off by the prospect of finding his penis bloodsmeared, he may welcome having a damp washcloth near the bed.

From time to time, women ask us for the Pill to eliminate their period. They're getting married or taking a second honeymoon and want supposedly carefree sex. We discourage this, explaining, "There's no reason to eliminate your period. What's more, the drug's not always effective, and you could suffer menstrual problems such as spotting and an irregular cycle."

* *Conception from sex during menses*

A patient claims she became pregnant as a result of having intercourse while she was menstruating. Is this possible?

Very much so. Sperm ejaculated into the vagina during menses may remain viable long enough to achieve fertilization after the woman ovulates. Advise your patients who want to avoid pregnancy to use contraception even when menstruating.

* *Postcoital vaginal burning before menses*

A few days before my period, I tend to experience postcoital vaginal burning. What's the explanation? What can I do about it?

The latter part of the menstrual cycle is dominated by progesterone, which can further engorge the vagina during the vasocongestion that arises from sexual stimulation. Orgasm may thus be accompanied by unfamiliar sensations, which you may experience as burning or other discomfort.

Sometimes all the remedy that's needed is a reinterpretation of these sensations; it might help to relax and accept them as normal, potentially pleasurable, and at worst extremely transient. If that doesn't work, a water-soluble lubricant may reduce the friction that increases discomfort. Also, circulation in the vaginal area can be improved by the Kegel exercise, which tones up the pubococcygeal muscle; whenever you urinate, stop the flow two or three times for about three seconds each time.

* *Tampon use from the start of menses*

Several girls aged 10, 11, and 12 are asking me whether they should use tampons. What should I tell them?

You can tell them it's a good idea. A girl who uses tampons is likely to become acquainted with her reproductive anatomy—and overcome any taboo about touching her genitalia. Moreover, her use of tampons tends to gradually stretch her hymen, which will ease her first intromission. Many girls also regard tampons as more esthetic than sanitary napkins; thus use of tampons often promotes a girl's adjustment to menarche.

To ease insertion of a tampon, we'd advise girls to use a water-soluble lubricant. Point out that the tampon should be inserted at an angle toward the small of the back, not upward as many girls think. Caution the girls against using deodorant tampons, which may cause an allergic reaction. Tell them, also, to insert fresh tampons fairly frequently throughout the day. For days of heaviest flow, you might suggest that the girls wear a tampon plus a minipad, the combination many young women find most acceptable.

It's also extremely important to put your instruction about tampons within the larger framework of sex education. These girls evidently are not being told much about sex at home and are looking to you for frank, thorough information. Almost certainly, they need to be taught the basics of the reproductive process. We've encountered adolescents who thought that using a tampon would mean they were no longer virgins.

In addition, these girls may have been influenced by the Biblical characterization of the menstruating woman as unclean (Leviticus 15:19–30). You can help them get off to a good start by presenting menstruation in as positive a light as possible. Volunteer favorable observations: "It's absolutely normal." "It's healthy and clean." "It's a sign of becoming a woman."

* *Solving primary amenorrhea*

My 15-year-old niece has never menstruated or grown pubic or axillary hair, although she has well-developed breasts. Her parents feel she's merely a "late developer" and are holding off taking her to a doctor. What do you advise?

By the time a girl reaches 15 or 16 without menstruating, we generally recommend a thorough evaluation to rule out endocrine disorders, ovarian diseases, chromosomal abnormalities, and drug or other problems that commonly cause primary amenorrhea.

For your niece, a prompt workup by a board-certified endocrinologist seems especially appropriate; her fully formed breasts in the absence of pubic and axillary hair are among signs suggestive of testicular feminization syndrome. This is a hereditary disorder in which a genetic male fetus fails to respond to testosterone and thus develops a vagina, clitoris, and labia (but no uterus or ovaries). The testes are in the abdomen or labia and produce estrogen that promotes development of the female physique.

The condition typically comes to light when a teenage girl presents with primary amenorrhea. It is sometimes diagnosed before puberty, if the testes cause a hernia or are palpable within the labia. It's generally advisable to remove the testes because they may become malignant. Also, if the testes are in the labia, they can cause painful coitus when the male partner thrusts against them. To permit comfortable intercourse, it may be necessary to lengthen the vagina, which tends to be about one-third shorter than normal.

Even if the syndrome is identified at birth, such children are properly reared as girls. Their insensitivity to testosterone makes their body build irreversibly female, and no adequate penis could be surgically created. Whether diagnosed or not, a girl with the syndrome usually has a normal childhood and is feminine in her self-image and behavior.

In counseling patients and their parents, it's imperative to reinforce the youngster's identity as a healthy female, avoiding the idea that the girl is really a boy. You might talk about a disorder involving the hormones made in the gonads, without mentioning such terms as "testes" and "male." To explain why fertility is impossible, it's truthful to say that the uterus has not developed normally. You may need to provide emotional support concerning marriage and adoption.

* *Amenorrhea in athletic women*

An 18-year-old girl who has been in intensive training with a track team has been amenorrheic for three years. What is the relationship between her athletic activity and her amenorrhea? Might she become sterile from atrophy of her reproductive organs? Does she require contraception despite her amenorrhea?

At least 10 percent of a female's body weight must be fat, or her estrogen will be too low for her to ovulate and menstruate. Thus amenorrhea is often found among otherwise normal women who are extremely lean—such as track team members, gymnasts, and ballet dancers.

In almost all cases, the amenorrhea is reversible. Soon after gaining the proper amount of weight, a woman will begin to menstruate, though it may take some months for her periods to regularize. Temporary amenorrhea that can be corrected by estrogens will not cause permanent atrophy.

However, three years is an unusually long time to be amenorrheic. We'd advise this young woman to undergo a complete endocrine evaluation. It would be prudent to rule out a pituitary adenoma or a prolactin-producing tumor.

Even if a fertile woman is amenorrheic, she requires contraception whenever she has intercourse, because ovulation can occur unpredictably.

* *Heavy menses following fundectomy*

About 10 years ago, I had surgery for removal of a Dalkon shield that had ruptured my uterine wall, embedded itself in the uterine fundus, and sawed through all but the last layer of small intestine. My gynecologist performed a tubal ligation and a fundectomy rather than a complete hysterectomy because, he said, he was concerned about my hormones. He also told me I'd have scant—if any—periods.

In fact, my periods have become a nightmare. They last five to seven days each month, with severe cramps. For two to four days, there's heavy bleeding and clotting that keeps me housebound. I'm only 35 years old, but I hope for an early change of life!

Physicians have been unable to tell me why this occurs, how there's enough uterine wall left for so much lining to develop, or what I can do about it. What's your opinion?

The fundectomy may have created scar tissue that acts as a foreign body, which can increase blood flow during menstruation. We'd suggest that you see a board-certified ob/gyn and get a diagnostic D&C or at least an endometrial biopsy, to rule out fibroids or such other causes of menorrhagia as endometrial hyperplasia, endometrial polyps, and early carcinoma of the endometrium. Pelvic sonography and hysteroscopy are other diagnostic procedures that could help establish the cause of your dysmenorrhea and excessive flow.

You also might consider having a complete hysterectomy, to remove the source of bleeding. The uterus actually has nothing to do with hormonal balance. It serves no purpose other than reproduction, which the tubal ligation has already precluded.

* *How to track menopause*

What's the most accurate way of telling when menopause is beginning? How long does the transition usually last?

You might advise patients to keep accurate records of their menstrual flows. The climacteric usually begins with changes in the menstrual cycle, with both longer and shorter intervals occurring between menses. Longer intervals gradually predominate and may last several months or a year or more until menstruation stops completely. One study has found that the mean duration of the climacteric is 6.3 years. One woman's transition time lasted a mere eight months; the most common was four years, and longest was 11 years.

See: Treloar AE. Records of menstrual flow held valuable in climacteric women. *Ob Gyn News* 16(20) 19, Oct 15, 1981

* *Contraception during menopause*

At age 51, after experiencing the signs of menopause, I stopped using contraception, only to become pregnant and miscarry. For how long should a perimenopausal woman continue using birth control? Which contraceptive method is considered best at her age?

It's advisable for a woman going through menopause to use contraception for a year following her last menstrual period. Ovulation can take place even after the beginning of reproductive senescence, with a much higher rate of fetal and maternal mortality than occurs in the usual childbearing years.

An IUD or diaphragm generally provides the best combination of effectiveness and safety for perimenopausal women. In this age group, the Pill poses too great a risk of cardiovascular and other side effects. Perimenopausal women are often good candidates for tubal coagulation, a simple sterilization method done through the navel via a laparoscope. Alternatively, male sex partners might undergo vasectomy.

* *Easing painful coitus after menopause*

A 53-year-old postmenopausal woman complains of painful intercourse. What's the probable cause? What's recommended?

If she has no psychosexual dysfunction or aversion to her partner, your patient may be suffering from atrophic (or senile) vaginitis, a degeneration of the vaginal mucosa caused by the decreased estrogen production that accompanies menopause. Vaginal lubrication diminishes, and a longer period of stimulation may be needed for the vaginal walls to moisten.

Further, with aging, the wall of the vagina loses some elasticity, and the vaginal barrel shrinks. The friction of intercourse may cause the vagina to crack and bleed. Reassure your patient that the condition is physiological. You may thus relieve any fears she may have of being sexually inadequate.

Estrogens administered vaginally via creams or suppositories often bring improvement—and cause fewer side effects than oral or parenteral estrogens. However, because even topical estrogens can be absorbed into the bloodstream, they should be used cautiously and should never be used by women with estrogen-dependent malignancies such as breast or endometrial cancer.

Graduated serial vaginal dilators may be recommended if your patient suffers from vaginal atrophy, especially if the introitus has tightened.

While atrophic vaginitis is the most common cause of painful intercourse for postmenopausal women, other possible causes of dyspareunia should, of course, be ruled out. Older women are more subject to uterine prolapse, cystocele, and rectocele. They are also more susceptible to vaginal and urinary tract infections and suffer a higher incidence of genitourinary neoplasms. To rule out possible organic causes of dyspareunia, it is mandatory that the patient be given a careful pelvic exam and a special Pap smear with maturation index, a cell count that reflects the amount of estrogen circulating in the blood.

CHAPTER 9

*

Sexually Transmitted Diseases

*

THE UNITED States is in the grip of an epidemic of sexually transmitted diseases. At any given time, 20 million Americans have syphilis, gonorrhea, or herpes. In addition, sexual contact can spread at least a dozen other types of infection.

The reservoir from which your patients might be infected is enormous. As contagious diseases, syphilis and gonorrhea are outranked in incidence only by the common cold. The number of new cases each year exceeds those of strep throat, scarlet fever, measles, mumps, hepatitis, and tuberculosis combined.

Be especially alert to sexually transmitted disease among young people. One person in five with gonorrhea is younger than 20. The rate of infection among 15- to 19-year-olds is rising faster than in any other age group.

Health professionals can best deal with this epidemic by treating a sexually transmitted disease as a health problem, not as a moral issue. It's important to provide treatment in as nonjudgmental a manner as possible. An accepting attitude is likely to encourage patients to seek early treatment on subsequent occasions.

Suspect that a patient with one sexually transmitted disease may have others as well, and perform appropriate tests. To ward off Ping-Pong reinfection, a steady sex partner may need to be treated at the same time as the patient with the presenting complaint. Otherwise, the partner may harbor the disease asymptomatically and thus may pass it on anew.

Urge patients with multiple sex partners to help protect themselves by using condoms. Also suggest periodic checkups to detect asymptomatic venereal disease.

* *Herpes in pregnancy*

An expectant mother in my prenatal course is worried about her herpes type II infection. Can it affect the fetus in utero? What precautions should be taken for delivery? How is the disease treated?

You can reassure your patient that the fetus in utero is probably safe. There's no direct evidence that herpesvirus crosses the placental barrier.

Still, there's at least a theoretical possibility that the virus *can* cause birth defects. Thus your patient would be wise to undergo amniocentesis, which could reveal a translocation of chromosomes, indicating a malformation. Unfortunately, some malformations may not show up in amniocentesis.

At delivery, the virus is a major hazard to infants, who have no immunity to it. A generalized infection typically leads to encephalitis, with death in eight out of 10 instances.

Telltale blisters anywhere on your patient's genitals call for a cesarean delivery. But even if there are no lesions, she still may have an active infection and, therefore, needs frequent Pap smears with a search for inclusion bodies. If these are present, she requires a follow-up viral culture. Only if all signs are negative can she risk a vaginal delivery.

There's no definitive treatment for herpes. Lesions take four to six weeks to heal, and can recur unpredictably. Large doses of the amino acid lysine (about 1,000 mg/day) appear to promote healing and retard recurrence, according to research reports. Recovery also seems to be speeded by contraceptive creams and foams containing nonoxynol-9 and by exposing the sores to fluorescent light and keeping them dry and aerated.

Caution your patient not to have intercourse for at least 10 days after her lesions heal—until then she may continue to transmit the infection. Remind her, also, to have a semiannual Pap smear; herpes appears to be associated with an increased incidence of cervical cancer. And let her know that you realize she's suffering from a painful, frustrating, frightening disease. With her added anxiety over her pregnancy, she needs emotional support—as well as a clear understanding of how she and the fetus are affected.

* *Can herpes spread via a heated rehab pool?*

A lifeguard who works in our heated rehabilitation pool has venereal herpes. Are patients at risk who swim in the pool with him? Also, he borrowed another guard's bathing suit. Can that person be sure the virus is dead if the suit has dried?

All parties seem safe from contracting the disease in the ways you describe. Herpesvirus doesn't survive in water at any temperature and thus can't be transmitted through the pool. Nor are clothes or other inanimate objects known to be vehicles of transmission; the virus doesn't survive outside of living cells.

* *Disease from toilet seats*

In public rest rooms, I see paper covers sold to make toilet seats more sanitary. What's the likelihood of an infection being spread by a toilet seat?

For intact tissues, very slight. According to the Centers for Disease Control, Atlanta, there's never been a documented case of a venereal or other disease being transmitted through perineal tissues or orifices by a contaminated toilet seat. Infective organisms that might gain entry through those sites don't ordinarily survive such a mode of transmission.

However, bacteria *can* culture on residues of feces, urine, and menstrual blood and infect exposed lesions. Avoiding direct contact with toilet seats therefore can't hurt and might well have hygienic value.

* *The dangers of "sleeping around"*

What are the risks associated with a sexually promiscuous lifestyle?

The more partners, the greater the chances of exposure to infection. The swinging lifestyle is thus definitely associated with a higher incidence of all sexually transmissible diseases. Both the male and female populations show increased rates of gonorrhea, syphilis, herpes, hepatitis B, pubic lice infestation, scabies, nongonococcal urethritis, lymphogranuloma venereum, genital warts, molluscum contagiosum, chancroid, and granuloma inguinale. Women, in addition, run an increased risk of cervical cancer, pelvic inflammatory disease, candidiasis, trichomoniasis, and *Haemophilus vaginalis* infections. Some of our patients have reported that they experienced psychological burnout from having sex with a lot of people, because they find the numerous shallow encounters ultimately depressing.

We generally refrain from using the word promiscuous, because it's usually interpreted as a derogatory term, a moral judgment against indiscriminate sex. In fact, people who have multiple sex partners are rarely undiscriminating, and even those who are extremely casual about their sexual encounters are entitled to their lifestyles. As health professionals, we're concerned about medical risks, while remaining nonjudgmental about the way patients choose to live.

* *Warts transmitted by sexual contact*

I assisted with the removal of warts from a patient's vulva and was told that this was probably a venereal disease. To what extent are warts transmitted sexually?

There's one type, called condylomata acuminata or anogenital warts, that occurs in moist areas, especially at the transition zone between mucous membrane and smooth, hairless (glabrous) skin. They appear as soft, pink, cauliflower-like growths at the anal border, on the glans penis, in the vulvar region, or at the corner of the mouth. Since they're frequently, though not necessarily, transmitted through close contact, caution patients against sexual activity until the warts have been removed. If a mouth lesion is involved, they should avoid kissing anybody.

Patients with perianal, periurethral, or vulvar warts should be examined internally for occult lesions. On anogenital mucous membranes, the growths can be treated by painting them with a thin coat of podophyllin solution (Podoben). Instruct the patient to wash off the chemical by bathing after four or five hours; treatments are repeated weekly until no new warts appear. Podophyllin is toxic and should be applied only by a physician. To prevent the patient from absorbing too much through his skin, extensive warts are reduced by excision or cryotherapy prior to treatment.

When anogenital warts arise on such glabrous areas as the shaft of the penis or the inner thighs, podophyllin won't work. These warts are usually removed with liquid nitrogen cryotherapy, with a vesicating agent such as cantharidin (Cantharone), or with a caustic or keratolytic agent such as salicylic acid (Calicylic, Duofilm, Keralyt). Whenever you see anogenital warts, it's important to screen the patient for gonorrhea and other sexually transmitted diseases that may be present as well.

See: Levine N. Recognizing and removing warts: New approaches to an age-old affliction. *Mod Med* 48:34 Dec 15, 1980, and Jan 15, 1981.

* *How to handle pubic lice*

I'm seeing many repeat cases of pubic lice. To what extent are they sexually transmitted? What do you recommend for treatment and prevention?

Most cases of pediculosis pubis are transmitted during sexual intercourse or other close physical contact. Pubic lice—also called crab lice or crabs—can also be spread via contaminated clothing, toilet seats, bedding, and the like. Continued contact with these objects—and with untreated family members and sex partners—can cause your patients to be reinfested.

To prevent recurrence, advise your patients to dry-clean or machine wash all clothes, bedding, and towels; items that can't be washed or cleaned, such as mattresses and pillows, should be treated with R & C Spray. Patients should also be alert to the signs of infestation in others. Teach them to suspect any intense itching, especially when the scratching results in infection or open sores. The crab louse inhabits not only the anogenital region, but also the short hairs of the underarms, eyebrows, eyelashes, chest, beard, and mustache.

Encourage your patients to play detective. Under a strong light and a magnifying lens, the louse looks like a grayish flake of dandruff attached to the thick hairs close to the skin. Louse eggs (nits) are usually firmly attached to the base of the hairs. Unlike dandruff flakes, nits adhere when brushed. Another clue to infestation: brown, dustlike louse excreta in the victim's underpants. There also may be gray-blue marks, 1 to 3 cm in diameter, on the trunk, thighs, and underarms—a systemic reaction to the lice's saliva.

The standard treatment begins with a hot soapy bath or shower, followed by an application of 1% gamma benzene hexachloride (Kwell) cream or lotion. Instruct your patient to wash the medication off after 12 to 24 hours, and to reapply it if needed, at weekly intervals. Warn the patient not to use turpentine, bug spray, or any other home remedy—all of which can cause rashes worse than the original problem.

When you see a case of crab lice, recommend a workup for other venereal diseases. Pediculosis pubis suggests a multiplicity of sex partners and is often accompanied by gonorrhea.

* Haemophilus vaginalis *Infections*

I'm seeing more and more patients with Haemophilus vaginalis *infections. Would you call it an epidemic? What's the preferred treatment?*

Chances are that most of the patients you're seeing are adolescent girls, since that group comprises the main reservoir of infection. Sexual intercourse is the primary mode of transmission, and the increased frequency you note is probably a reflection of the increase in coitus among teenagers and could not be considered an epidemic.

You can recognize *H. vaginalis* infection by the gray, often frothy discharge it causes, sometimes accompanied by mild itching. A foul odor suggests a co-existing *Candida* infection. Treatment usually includes ampicillin PO or tetracycline PO, or by suppository. To avoid an overgrowth of *Candida*, nystatin (Mycostatin, Nilstat) vaginal suppositories may be prescribed. Vaginal sulfonamide creams (Sultrin, Vagitrol) and suppositories may be less effective against *H. vaginalis*, but don't cause candidiasis.

* *Trichomoniasis and male sterility*

A 22-year-old male, in the hospital for a sports injury, asked if a long period of untreated trichomonal infection would have caused permanent damage to his sperm ducts, possibly leading to infertility. He and his girlfriend have apparently had the infection for some time, and are now being treated with metronidazole (Flagyl).

This young man may have suffered urethritis and prostatitis from the neglected infection and may be worried about that. You can reassure him that he'll probably have no significant sequelae; *Trichomonas* does not invade the germinal epithelium or cause scarring of the collecting ducts.

You should warn patients with trichomoniasis, however, not to drink alcohol while taking metronidazole. An interaction can cause abdominal distress, nausea, vomiting, flushing, and headache. Patients taking metronidazole should also immediately report any neurological symptoms (dizziness, lack of coordination, ataxia, and the like); the drug can lead to persistent peripheral neuropathy, marked by numbness or paresthesia of an extremity.

Be especially watchful when patients are taking metronidazole concurrently with coumarin (Dicumarol) or warfarin (Coumadin, Panwarfin). The drug potentiates the anticoagulants' effects, prolonging prothrombin time. It also may flatten T-waves in ECG tracings.

* *Gonorrhea: follow-up care for female patients*

A woman showing a severe onset of gonorrhea—dysuria, frequency, vaginal discharge—has been treated with penicillin and probenecid. What's the advisable follow-up? Is it sufficient to make sure she's asymptomatic?

Abatement of symptoms is not sufficient assurance that a woman's gonococcal infection has been eradicated. Gonorrhea in a woman is nearly always asymptomatic. And even if she initially shows severe symptoms, the infection may become silent after treatment.

From seven to 14 days after completion of treatment, she, therefore, should undergo a culture of both the endocervical and anal canals, even if only one was infected. Gonococci are fragile, so to ensure a reliable result the culture needs to be obtained and incubated with extreme care. A suitable medium (such as modified Thayer-Martin) is required. A negative culture indicates a cure.

There are other ways, but this evaluation is the best available. By contrast, a gram-stained smear, while quicker, can yield both false positives and false negatives.

* *Is there an "incurable" gonorrhea?*

Patients are asking me about an "incurable" Vietnamese gonorrhea that's supposedly spreading across this country. How much truth is there to the rumor?

Very little. They've probably heard scare stories about strains of gonococci that do resist even high levels of penicillin and tetracycline. Some of these strains evidently were picked up by GIs in Southeast Asia.

You can assure patients, however, that other drugs are effective against such organisms. A 2-gm intramuscular injection of spectinomycin (Trobicin) is the recommended alternative. If that doesn't work, the infection can generally be treated parenterally with cefoxitin (Mefoxin) or possibly orally with trimethoprim-sulfamethoxazole (Bactrim, Septra).

It's important that patients realize that such resistant infections are rare. The typical case of gonorrhea can be cured with a single dose of procaine penicillin G plus probenecid. The last thing we need in the current gonorrhea epidemic is for patients to stay away from clinics in the belief they can't be cured of the disease.

* *Persistent urethritis after gonorrhea*

After being treated for gonorrhea and showing negative cultures for the disease, a patient continues to have a discharge from his penis and burning discomfort during urination. What could be the cause? How should it be treated?

Chances are he has nongonococcal urethritis (NGU), which often occurs along with gonorrhea and produces many of the same symptoms. In men, these can include a mucopurulent penile discharge, dysuria, and occasional hematuria. Women are usually asymptomatic, but may experience cystitis, dysuria, vaginal discharge, abdominal pain, or cervicitis with inflammatory erosion.

NGU is actually the most common sexually transmitted disease, occurring about twice as often as gonorrhea. The major cause is *Chlamydia trachomatis*, a bacteria-like organism that thrives as an intracellular parasite and is resistant to penicillin. Oral tetracycline or erythromycin usually clears up the infection in a week. Cervicitis necessitates a Pap smear and, occasionally, cryosurgery. The infection may recur within two to six weeks, depending on the organism's life-cycle phase at the time of initial treatment.

Chlamydial NGU is generally diagnosed empirically when microscopic studies of discharge samples show pus cells in the absence of gonorrhea. If untreated, the disease can cause men to develop potentially sterilizing epididymitis. Women may experience pelvic inflammatory disease and salpingitis, with a high risk of tubal pregnancy. Neonates infected while passing through the birth canal often develop conjunctivitis (inclusion blennorrhea) and chlamydial pneumonia. It's therefore prudent to check for chlamydia early in pregnancy and again several weeks prior to vaginal delivery.

* *False positives with syphilis tests*

For the past 21 years, since I was 11 years old, I've had false positive VDRL tests for syphilis, even though I've been negative for all the conditions that can cause a positive result. Throughout my nursing career, hospitals have accepted this anomaly as one of those things that can occur. Recently however, I applied for a position in an ICU and, in the physical, took not only a VDRL but also an FTA-ABS test, which is supposed to be specific for syphilis.

To my horror, both tests showed positive. The hospital said it would hire me if I took the appropriate penicillin therapy. I received the maximum dosage recommended for late, latent syphilis, but my tests remained positive.

I concluded that I must have had untreated syphilis for all these years and thus must have suffered neurological damage. I, therefore, had a lumbar puncture performed. My CSF was normal, but my tests, repeated at three-month intervals, remain positive. I've found it impossible to get a hospital job until I can prove that I'm syphilis-free and I feel humiliated and confused. Why do my tests show these positive results? How can I convince hospitals that I'm not a hazard to patients?

Officials at the Venereal Disease Control Division of the Centers for Disease Control, Atlanta, speculate that you're one of hundreds of thousands of people who have an idiosyncratic reaction to the VDRL (Venereal Disease Research Laboratory) test, which is a screening procedure that demonstrates the presence of a reagin. The test may show a false positive if the patient is pregnant or has a rheumatologic disease such as rheumatoid arthritis or systemic lupus erythematosus. False positives also may be caused by the common cold, influenza, mononucleosis, hepatitis, malaria, leprosy, and other infections as well as by many drugs, notably oral contraceptives and heroin. Even in the absence of any of these, the test can show positive in some individuals, as is evidently your case.

Your positive FTA-ABS (fluorescent treponemal antibody absorption) results may have come from subjective errors in the lab. Especially when a VDRL is positive, microscopists have a tendency to overread FTA-ABS slides. We've seen patients who were actually syphilis-free reported as high as 2+ (out of 4+).

What's puzzling is why any hospital would think you'd be contagious. Possibly the personnel you've dealt with have the same prejudices against syphilis that many laymen do. In fact, the disease can be transmitted only in the primary and secondary stages, which generally pass within three years. Even if you had late, latent syphilis, you'd be unable to infect patients.

We'd suggest you get in touch with a venereologist. Your local health department can probably tell you of one near you. Such a specialist would be in a position to have your tests conducted accurately and to draft a persuasive document you can show potential employers.

* *Cured syphilis and positive test reactions*

My fiance was treated for syphilis during the Vietnam War with the maximum dosage of penicillin and was pronounced cured. However, every Kahn test he's undergone since has been weakly positive. Our doctor says this is "almost like negative," but I'm not completely convinced. Is there any risk in our getting married?

Probably not. After being cured of syphilis, some people have an immunologic aberration that produces a positive reaction, even though there are no live spirochetes. To be absolutely certain, however, we'd suggest your fiance undergo a definitive Treponema pallidum immobilization (TPI) serologic test. This test should preferably be done by a venereologist.

* A syphilitic chancre on the finger

I saw a woman who had a punched-out sore on her finger. Could it have been a syphilitic chancre?

Indeed so. Primary syphilis, which appears about three weeks after exposure, begins with small, fluid-filled lesions that erode into sores with hard raised edges and clear bases. These chancres usually erupt in and around the genitals, mouth, or anus—wherever the spirochetes first entered the body. But the lesions may also occur on fingers, nipples, and eyelids.

Because they're usually painless and disappear in three to six weeks, chancres on nongenital sites are commonly assumed to be simple sores. A chancre on the finger is thus particularly treacherous because, if treated as an ordinary sore, it can spread the infection to any mucous membrane it comes in contact with.

* Lesions that mimic syphilitic ulcers

Three months ago, a patient presented with symptoms much like those of primary syphilis. He had ulcers on the penis, with redness of the glans; the foreskin showed two small ulcers and edema. However, we could obtain no microscopic or serologic evidence of a syphilitic infection; nor did cultures grow herpesvirus. The lesions resolved without treatment. Now the patient is back with an identical condition. Can you suggest what might be causing it?

It could be a fixed drug eruption, in which lesions occur at the same site after the patient takes a particular drug or one that's chemically similar. The typical lesion begins as a dusky erythema. Edema of the dermis leads to blisters, which often open. Since the genital mucosa are frequently involved, the clinical picture may mimic syphilis. The lesions don't necessarily follow every contact with one drug, so the patient may not be aware of the connection.

A detailed drug history can help you pinpoint the cause of the eruption. Sulfonamides are frequent offenders; fixed genital drug eruptions were also linked recently to trimethoprim-sulfamethoxazole (Bactrim, Septra) Other causes are the laxative phenolphthalein (Alophen, Ex-Lax), barbiturates, tetracycline, salicylates, quinine, phenylbutazone (Azolid, Butazolidin), and oxyphenbutazone (Oxalid, Tandearil).

It's important to warn the patient to avoid all preparations containing the offending agent. The fixed drug eruption is a clear sign of drug sensitivity, which can take more severe forms with subsequent exposures.

See: Talbot MD. Fixed genital drug eruption. *Practitioner* 224:823, 1980.

CHAPTER 10

*

Contraception

*

A WIDE VARIETY of birth control methods have been used over the ages. Medical science is still seeking a perfectly safe, perfectly effective contraceptive.

In giving contraceptive advice, impress upon your patients that all methods but one have some potential for failure or side effects. The only 100 percent safe and effective method of contraception is abstinence.

Also let them know that no single contraceptive method is right for everyone. Any choice of contraceptive should involve consideration of these points: the protection the method affords, the risk of adverse reactions, and the method's suitability to an individual's preferences, health history, religious convictions, and the frequency and circumstances of sexual activity.

In counseling patients, emphasize contraception as a shared responsibility. Particularly in dealing with teenage patients, let them know that if a couple can't talk about contraception and jointly decide on a suitable method—then they almost certainly aren't ready for the responsibilities of sexual intercourse.

* *How to prevent condom failure*

A patient maintains that her boyfriend has consistently worn a condom during intercourse. Nevertheless, she's pregnant. How fragile are condoms? How can they be kept from breaking?

American-made condoms are thin but tough; they're manufactured under strict FDA standards and generally break only if they dry out from age or are subjected to heat or other abuse. For maximum shelf life, it's wise to store condoms in a refrigerator; at room temperature, an unopened packet is safe for about a year. Keeping condoms in a pocket, wallet, or glove compartment causes rapid deterioration. It's wise to buy condoms from a store, instead of a machine, which may have old merchandise.

Condoms that are lubricated in their packages are least likely to break from dryness. For do-it-yourself lubrication, a surgical or spermicidal jelly is best; petroleum jelly or oils can cause the condom to deteriorate. Patients should examine a condom before using it, but avoid needless stretching or inflating, which may damage it. Of course, if there's any question whatever about a condom's safety, it should be thrown away and a new one used.

Your patient's pregnancy may not have resulted from the condom's breaking, however. The condom may have slipped off partially or completely inside her vagina as the penis shrank after ejaculation, permitting leakage of semen. A male wearing a condom should therefore withdraw his penis before it softens, securing the condom by holding his fingers around its base. Because sperm can migrate from outside the body into the vagina, he should move away from his partner and only then unroll the condom and wipe his penis. A condom is a good but not a perfect contraceptive; for optimal protection it should be used with foam or a diaphragm.

* *Condoms and interrupted lovemaking*

Many of the men we counsel in the family planning clinic where I work object to using condoms because they say that putting them on interrupts lovemaking. Any suggestions?

The men may be afraid of losing their erections during the so-called interruption. This is less likely to happen if fitting a condom over the erect penis is made an exciting part of sex play, with the female partner assisting. To add to the sensuousness of condoms, the partners might enjoy using a variety of designs and colors.

It's a good idea for a man to practice putting on a condom alone; there's a minimal amount of technique involved in unrolling it and keeping it from entangling pubic hair. A lubricated prerolled condom with a reservoir tip to catch the semen is generally the easiest kind to put on; if the condom doesn't have a reservoir, a half-inch should be left loose at the end for this purpose.

* *Dealing with complaints that condoms lessen pleasure*

What can I tell teenage boys who argue that condoms reduce the sensation of intercourse? They say, "It's like shaking hands wearing a rubber glove," and refuse to use this excellent contraceptive method.

Males who seek greater sensitivity often find satisfaction with condoms made from lambskin or extra-thin latex. They also may experience a range of sensations by using condoms embossed with various textures. You might mention to teenagers that many adults find such a decrease in sensitivity to be an advantage, because it may somewhat delay ejaculation and thus prolong the act for the enhanced pleasure of both partners.

* *Convincing boys to use condoms*

How can I encourage sexually active teenage boys to use condoms? They're often unmoved when I point out that this is an effective means of birth control and can protect them against many sexually transmitted diseases.

A teenager who won't use contraceptives isn't accepting responsibility for his capacity to cause pregnancy. Often he refuses to consider the fact of his fertility and so he doesn't do anything to control it. Moreover, boys often feel pressured to have intercourse; they worry about their performance, and anxiety keeps them from taking sensible precautions. We've seen pregnancies caused by boys who had condoms in their wallets but weren't able emotionally to deal with the ramifications of their sexual desire.

We've found it helpful to reassure adolescents that, though their sexual impulses are perfectly healthy, they embody the awesome power to create new life and that this is a fact that can never be ignored. As with any form of power, there's a need to control it. Condoms provide the best contraceptive method for most teenagers: They're nearly foolproof, especially if used with foam or a diaphragm. They have virtually no side effects. They offer good protection against infection. They're inexpensive. They're widely available. They require no prescription. And they're easily carried in a pocket or purse.

Alas, you're up against the characteristic shortsightedness of adolescence, so we'd suggest putting your warnings and advice in specific terms that a boy can apply to himself right now. Birth control is an abstraction that may not mean much to a teenager, but he'll probably take notice if you spell out the problems he's likely to encounter if he gets someone pregnant. If he's having intercourse with a steady girlfriend, you might appeal to his manly concern for her.

In explaining what you mean by protection against disease, some graphic details may prove most convincing. Disease is a vague word; but the threat of penile burning, foul discharge, and urethral stricture leaves little to the imagination. A few words on the consequences of gonococcal arthritis, endocarditis, and meningitis might help as well.

Teenagers often complain that condoms are difficult to obtain or that they're afraid to buy them. They're generally most comfortable buying the product in a large discount department store, where condoms are likely to be on display. Some teenagers believe it's against the law for them to buy condoms; actually, the Supreme Court has ruled that sale of contraceptives to minors is perfectly legal.

* *What to advise for teenage contraception*

What contraceptive would you recommend for a teenage girl?

That depends on how often she has intercourse—and how likely she is to plan ahead for it.

Most teenagers have intercourse infrequently and are short on foresight. (In fact, many teenage girls feel guilty about deliberately planning sex.) We find that contraceptive foam plus a condom is the best method for them. The materials are inexpensive, widely available, and require no prescription. And the method is extremely effective, with no side effects.

Furthermore, the condom provides protection against venereal disease, which is epidemic among teenagers. It also requires the boy to share responsibility for avoiding pregnancy. Having both parties face that possibility makes it more likely that contraception will be used. We make a point of telling young female patients, "If a boy won't wear a condom, he's not mature enough to have intercourse with."

A diaphragm with a condom is even more effective and is equally free of side effects. But this method is suited mainly to mature young women who can be counted on to use it properly. And unless the patient has intercourse frequently, it may not be worth the investment in money and time. We never consider a diaphragm for an immature girl with a helter-skelter sex life. Such girls are rarely able to cope with the equipment, the modest skill required for insertion, or the discipline needed.

For a girl who has frequent intercourse but isn't likely to use either a condom with foam or a diaphragm reliably, an IUD may be the best contraceptive, as it provides passive compliance. Although somewhat less effective than the Pill, IUDs cause no systemic side effects. The cramps that often accompany the first few months' use of the IUD, however, may be difficult for some adolescent girls to tolerate, so they require reassurance that the cramping will decrease.

Most teenagers can tolerate copper-containing IUDs such as the nulliparous Copper T or Cu-7, which are smaller than the plastic devices. Unlike plastic IUDs, which can stay in place indefinitely, a copper device must be replaced every two or three years.

* *Resistance to contraceptive advice*

As part of the counseling I give in an abortion facility, I review birth control methods. Occasionally, a young patient refuses to discuss contraception, insisting she has no desire for another sexual relationship. Taking into account the emotional trauma she's experiencing, how would you advise her?

We'd suggest she come back in three weeks. By then, her initial trauma over the abortion is likely to be resolved, and she'll have seen that life goes on pretty much as before. At that time, she may be ready to accept the fact that sooner or later she'll need contraception.

To promote a healthier sexual attitude, you might help her distinguish between abortion and other aspects of sexuality. She may need more than one counseling session before she realizes that sexual feelings need not necessarily lead to coitus or pregnancy or abortion.

It's also extremely important to support her if she continues her resolve to remain abstinent. We've found that many young postabortion patients are, in fact, not ready for another relationship involving intercourse. To counteract peer pressures, we help them rehearse saying, "I don't want to," with no apologies or explanations. We also impress upon them that there's a wide range of sexual options not involving intercourse. If she's involved in a relationship with one person, it may be helpful to include him in the counseling sessions.

* *Using a diaphragm safely*

How long before intercourse can a woman insert her diaphragm? For how long afterward should she wear it? How long does one last?

First, emphasize to your patients that the diaphragm is but one part of a contraceptive system. Before inserting it, the woman needs to spread about a teaspoonful of spermicidal jelly or cream on the saucerlike inner surface and the rim. Otherwise, sperm can get around the device and make her pregnant.

The diaphragm will provide protection if it's inserted within the two hours before the woman has intercourse. If more than two hours elapse between insertion and intercourse she'll be safest if she leaves the device in place but inserts more spermicide: cream, jelly, foam , or a suppository. Each such application protects her against the sperm in one ejaculation. Before every additional coitus, she needs to insert another dose of spermicide.

You can add the caution that it's not a good idea to interrupt sex play to insert the diaphragm. Sexual arousal changes the location of the cervix, raising the risk of an improper fit. If your patient thinks she might possibly have intercourse while she's out on a date, she can insert her diaphragm before going out and later insert an applicatorful of spermicide, if it's needed.

Warn your patient to keep the diaphragm in place—and not to douche—for at least six hours after intercourse. She can wear the diaphragm for days without adverse effect. Earlier removal, however, allows the vagina to cleanse itself and reduces the risk of irritation and infection.

With good care, your patient can expect her diaphragm to last for about two years. Advise her to wash it with mild soap and warm water, then air-dry it and dust it with cornstarch before replacing it in its case. Suggest she check it after each use for weak spots and pinholes, gently pulling the rubber away from the rim while she holds the diaphragm against a bright light.

Remind your patient that she may need a change in diaphragm size if she loses or gains more than 20 pounds or if she has been pregnant since her last fitting. Here are some warning signals that her diaphragm size or her insertion technique is faulty: The diaphragm causes her discomfort; it's no longer snug; she can easily place a finger between its rim and the recess of her vaginal wall; her partner can feel it; there's blood on it when she's not menstruating.

Recommend that she have her diaphragm and insertion technique checked every year, during her annual gynecological exam. Even women who've used diaphragms for many years often grow careless about them.

* Bathing with a diaphragm in place

If a woman is using a diaphragm plus contraceptive jelly, how soon after having intercourse may she swim or take a bath?

Immediately, because water usually doesn't enter the vagina. The organ is not a cavity, as is commonly believed; the soft walls fold into each other filling the lumen. *Forcible* entry of water, however, can indeed compromise the spermicide; it's therefore advisable to warn patients not to douche and to keep the diaphragm in place for at least six hours after intercourse.

* *Contraception and underwater lovemaking*

Can a woman using a diaphragm plus contraceptive jelly have intercourse in a tub or pool without risking pregnancy?

Afraid not. When a woman bathes or swims, water doesn't usually enter the vagina because the soft walls fold into each other, filling the lumen. But, during coitus immersed in water, the thrusting penis can pump water into the vagina, dislodging the diaphragm and flushing out the contraceptive jelly. The water can also wash away normal vaginal lubrication and introduce chlorine, soap, or microorganisms that may cause vaginitis. In general, we've concluded that making love under water has a better press than it deserves.

* *What to advise about IUDs*

What can I tell patients about the pros and cons of the IUD? How does the device prevent pregnancy? What are the side effects? Is it an abortifacient?

Nonmedicated IUDs such as the Lippes Loop and the Saf-T-Coil appear to act primarily by stimulating an inflammatory reaction in the endometrium, so that macrophages and other cells will engulf the sperm or ovum. It is also likely that IUDs speed up passage of the ovum through the fallopian tube and interfere with the implantation of the fertilized ovum in the uterine wall.

In the Cu-7 and Tatum-T IUDs, copper wire coiled around the devices increases the inflammatory reaction and is also toxic to sperm. In the Progestasert IUD, a reservoir of progesterone keeps the endometrium in a pregnancy-like state, making implantation unlikely.

As far as effectiveness goes, the IUD is generally ranked second to the Pill. Its other major advantage is that it requires no preparation prior to intercourse; this not only permits spontaneous sex but also provides passive protection for women who are unlikely to take, or are mentally incapable of taking, active measures.

Warn your patients that IUD users are one-and-a-half to five times more likely than nonusers to develop pelvic inflammatory disease (PID), which may interfere with future fertility. Most at risk are nulliparous women under age 25, women with histories of PID, and women who have more than one sex partner or who frequently change partners. The ideal candidate for an IUD is thus an older woman with just one sex partner and no desire for a future pregnancy.

Among women with IUDs who do become pregnant, there is an increased incidence of ectopic pregnancy. A rare complication is perforation of the uterus, usually during insertion. Especially during the first three to six months of use, menstrual bleeding may be heavier and there may be bleeding and cramping between periods.

Technically, IUDs can be considered abortifacients in that they may act against a fertilized ovum, causing it to be expelled should it become implanted. It's important to tell patients of such effects. Women who are opposed to abortion may want to use another method of contraception; conversely, other women may feel reassured that, with an IUD, even if fertilization does take place it is not likely to result in a term pregnancy (although some IUD pregnancies have reached term).

Teach patients with IUDs how to check for the device's string after each menstrual period. While it's unlikely that expulsion of the device would go unnoticed, the IUD could be downwardly displaced, so that the tip of the device is palpable—leaving the patient vulnerable to pregnancy. To help patients become comfortable with touching the vagina, give them a guided tour of their genitalia with the aid of a mirror. For added protection, suggest that they also use contraceptive foam during the most fertile days of their menstrual cycles.

The IUD is contraindicated in the presence of pregnancy, pelvic infection, congenital anomalies of the uterus, and severe cervical stenosis. Other contraindications include severe uterine retroflexion and a uterine cavity distorted by fibroids. Severe anemia, undiagnosed vaginal bleeding, and coagulation disorders or the use of anticoagulant drugs also usually make an IUD unsuitable. In addition, the device poses an unacceptable danger of infection to women with valvular heart disease (who are at risk of bacterial endocarditis); women using immunosuppressive agents, including corticosteroids; and women with diseases that suppress normal immunity, such as leukemia and lymphoma.

* The Pill and decreased desire

A patient who's recently gone on the Pill complains of diminished interest in sex. Is there a connection?

Very possibly. Decreased libido is a fairly common side effect of oral contraceptives. Women on the Pill widely report a waning of sexual desire, with corresponding difficulty in arousal.

If the oral contraceptive causes merely a slowing of sexual response, a longer period of stimulation may suffice to correct the problem. Many women, however, need to weigh the advantages of the Pill against the disadvantages of being dysfunctional. Switching to an OC of a different formulation is worth a try. Varying the proportion of estrogen may be beneficial, or the change may have a placebo effect.

* Early use of the Pill after abortion

To reduce the risk of thromboembolism, the abortion clinic where I work postpones prescribing oral contraceptives until the patient's first postabortion menstrual period. However, many patients don't return for their routine exam and resume intercourse without adequate protection. Would it be safe to start them on OCs earlier?

It would seem so. Finnish investigators have found that patients can start taking oral contraceptives one week after a first-trimester abortion without increasing their risk of developing thromboemboli. This allows a clinic such as yours to write a prescription at the time of the visit, with appropriate near-term instructions about when to start the Pill. During that first postabortion week, the patient generally won't be ovulating and so is at no risk of conception if she has intercourse without protection. The investigators also found that an IUD can be safely inserted at the end of the abortion procedure, so the patient leaves with automatic contraception.

See: Lahteenmaki P, Rasi V, Luukkainen T, et al. Coagulation factors in women using oral contraceptives or intrauterine contraceptive devices immediately after abortion. *Am J Obstet Gynecol* 141:175, 1981.

* Age and the Pill

One of my patients has been taking oral contraceptives since they were first introduced in the '60s. She's had no ill effects, but could she be getting too old to use the Pill safely?

Yes. A woman older than 35 who uses the Pill is at elevated risk of cardiovascular complications such as myocardial infarction or stroke.

This is especially true if she smokes. For example, an OC user who consumes 25 or more cigarettes a day has 39 times the normal risk of a heart attack. In addition, with increasing age, she might have hypertension or diabetes, which would further increase the risk of heart attack. We'd suggest she consult her doctor about another form of contraception. However, if she has no risk factors (smoking, hypertension, diabetes, or hyperlipoproteinuria) and no other contraceptive method is appropriate, then consideration can be given to continuing OC use.

* *Timing conception after using OCs*

After taking oral contraceptives for 10 years, a patient now wants to conceive. When in her menstrual cycle should she stop taking the Pill? How long should she remain off the drug before trying to conceive? Could the cumulative effects of the Pill's hormones damage the fetus or result in defects not detectable at birth?

We'd recommend that the patient go off the Pill at the time of her next menses. She should then wait at least three months before attempting to become pregnant, meanwhile obtaining protection from an alternative form of contraception such as a diaphragm or a condom plus foam. This interval is advisable because there's an increased incidence of miscarriages in pregnancies that occur immediately following cessation of oral contraceptives. Other than this, you can reassure your patient that there are no reports of the Pill's affecting the fetus or causing birth defects.

* *Effect of antibiotics on the Pill*

After taking oral contraceptives for many years without difficulty, a patient has accidentally become pregnant. Conception apparently occurred while she was undergoing tetracycline therapy for sinusitis. Do you think the antibiotic could have neutralized the contraceptive?

Very possibly. Failure of oral contraceptives has been linked to tetracycline (Achromycin, Panmycin, Sumycin) and such other antibiotics as ampicillin (Amcill, Omnipen), chloramphenicol (Chloromycetin), and rifampin (Rifadin, Rifamate, an ingredient in Rimactane).

It's thought that the antibiotics inactivate contraceptive steroids by increasing their metabolic breakdown in the liver or by killing intestinal bacteria whose enzymes may be responsible for reactivating the steroids once they've been metabolized.

Thus, a woman who is taking both an oral contraceptive and an antibacterial would be safest during intercourse if she used an additional contraceptive method, especially if she's taking a low-dose estrogen product (e.g., Brevicon, Demulen 1/35, Modicon).

See: Andersen RC and Davis LJ. Antibiotic-oral contraceptive interaction? *Drug Intel Clin Pharm* 15:280, 1981.

* *Contraceptive foam and birth defects*

A resident in my hospital says that contraceptive foam can cause birth defects. Is this true?

A link hasn't been conclusively established. The doctor is probably referring to a study of mothers who, in the 10 months before conceiving, used a contraceptive foam, gel, or cream containing nonoxynol 9 or octoxynol (contained in Emko, Koromex, Ortho, and many other spermicidal products). Infants born to such women suffered twice the control group's rate of congenital disorders, chiefly neoplasms, hypospadias, limb deformities, and syndromes associated with chromosomal abnormalities.

Investigators speculate that the spermicidal ingredients might damage sperm or be absorbed through the vaginal membranes, leading to birth defects.

However, the researchers carefully point out that the study "leaves a number of important questions unanswered." For example, the absence of a single, well-defined syndrome among the infants raises doubt about a causal connection between the spermicides and the birth defects. In addition, since the study was conducted long after the contraceptives were used, the precise time of exposure has not been established. Therefore, conclude the investigators, the results "should be considered tentative until confirmed by other data."

See: Jick H, Walker AM, Rothman KJ, et al: Vaginal spermicides and congenital disorders. *JAMA* 245:1329, 1981.

* *Contraceptive suppositories*

Patients occasionally ask me about the effectiveness of the contraceptive suppositories that are heavily advertised to the public. What's your evaluation of them?

When our female patients want an over-the-counter contraceptive, we advise them to use spermicidal foam, not a suppository. For maximum effectiveness, either product also requires that a condom be used.

We prefer foam because it provides a more reliable barrier. Suppositories are intended to melt or effervesce and form a shield. However, they may fail to melt adequately at body temperature. And if the vagina is dry, they may fail to effervesce.

Foam also seem less likely to interrupt sex play. It can be inserted up to an hour before coitus. By contrast, some suppositories are less convenient, because they must be inserted a mere 10 to 15 minutes prior to intromission.

✻ Pros and cons of sterilization

What pros and cons should I mention to patients regarding vasectomy or tubal ligation as a form of birth control?

The positive points are that both these methods have low failure rates (about one in 1,000), pose only a one-time risk, and have minimal side effects following the surgical recovery. Several recent studies indicate that vasectomy in monkeys increases the likelihood of their developing atherosclerosis. But no evidence of this effect has been uncovered in men, and the procedure is still generally regarded as safe (as is tubal ligation).

The disadvantage is that the procedures are reversible in only 60 to 70 percent of patients, even using advanced microsurgical techniques. Thus they may prematurely foreclose patients' options for having children.

✻ Can a vasectomy lead to a heart attack

Several women asked me if a man's having a vasectomy could cause him to suffer a heart attack. It seems that a physician on a TV talk show said it could. These women, whose husbands have had vasectomies, are worried. Is there any truth to the MD's statement?

It might be true if the patient's cardiovascular functioning is already so compromised that the surgery adds an unsupportable stress. The doctor might, in fact, have been pointing out the need for a physical exam prior to a vasectomy to rule out that risk.

A patient who feels emasculated by the surgery might also be at risk. The resulting emotional stress could conceivably precipitate a heart attack in a vulnerable man—but it's not terribly likely.

Alternatively, the doctor might have been referring to a study of monkeys that showed a tendency toward atherosclerosis following vasectomy. This is possibly related to the increased titers of antibodies formed in response to the trapped sperm. But at present, there's no hard evidence linking vasectomy to atherosclerosis or heart attack in man.

Suffice it to say that any vasectomy candidate should be given a physical exam beforehand. Assure him that his output of male hormones won't decrease, that he'll be able to ejaculate as before, and that he need feel no loss of masculinity.

He should also know that he's likely to have pain and swelling for several days post-op, which he can relieve with ice packs. Supporting the scrotum with a folded towel draped across the upper thighs, while the patient lies in bed, may also help.

CHAPTER 11

*

Fertility and Infertility

*

INFERTILITY AFFECTS about one in eight U.S. couples of childbearing age. Couples are considered infertile when pregnancy has not occurred after a year of sexual relations without the use of birth control. Encourage such patients to consult a specialist in infertility.

With treatment, perhaps half of infertile couples may be able to conceive. New treatments—pharmacology, laser microsurgery, in vitro fertilization—make pregnancy a greater possibility than ever before.

In counseling infertile couples, be aware that sexual problems may arise from their attempts at conceiving. Having to make love by the calendar is likely to add tension to an already stressful situation. In focusing on achieving pregnancy, couples often lose sight of the pleasurable aspects of lovemaking. Common problems include impotence, decreased sexual desire, and inability to reach orgasm. Both partners may bring to the sexual relationship feelings of guilt, blame, depression, inadequacy, and anger.

It's best for couples trying to conceive to be as spontaneous in their sex lives as they can manage. As far as possible, they should try to concentrate on the pleasures of sex rather than on its intended goal. Ideally, temperature charts and other intrusive diagnostic tests are put aside as soon as they've served their purpose.

Many couples find self-help groups an excellent tool for venting their feelings about fertility problems. For information about support groups for infertile couples, contact Resolve Inc., P.O. Box 474, Belmont, Mass. 02178.

* A case of possible infertility

After laparoscopy, an infertile woman's doctor diagnosed her as having moderate endometriosis; a left ovarian cyst, probably endometrial; and mild chronic salpingitis. He started her on danazol (Danocrine). Evidently he told her that surgery might be necessary despite the risk of scarring and adhesions, that there was nothing he could do for the salpingitis, and that the tubes were open and perfused easily but that the environment on the inside was incompatible with fertilization.

Now the woman has come to me in confusion over the doctor's remarks. Can you explain what they might mean? What should I advise? The patient wants to know if anything can be done for salpingitis, how she got it, what her chances are of ever getting pregnant, and so on.

Such questions really need careful answering by a physician who's familiar with your patient. We don't know, for example, what's causing the salpingitis. It could be secondary to endometriosis, which tends to interfere with pregnancy regardless of its extent (and that may have given rise to the doctor's reported remark about an environment that's "incompatible with fertilization"). On the other hand, salpingitis may be part of generalized pelvic inflammatory disease, and its origin may be bacterial, viral, mycoplasmal, or even tuberculous.

It's consistent with good medical practice to treat endometriosis with a three- to nine-month course of danazol, at which time another laparoscopy may be indicated. If your patient is then not satisfied with the care she's receiving, she ought to get a second opinion from an infertility specialist.

Meanwhile, of course, she should have her questions answered by her current doctor. Infertility often causes patients great emotional distress; when receiving a diagnosis, they frequently fail to register essential information or ask important questions. You might suggest that she and her husband write down every question they have and then discuss them at a special appointment with her physician. You can assure the couple that most specialists welcome such consultations.

* Reduced fertility from loss of an ovary

After undergoing unilateral oophorectomy, a patient has asked me how much the surgery will reduce her normal monthly ovulation and her prospects for pregnancy. Will she continue to menstruate every month? How will birth control pills affect her remaining ovary?

If your patient formerly menstruated once every four weeks, she's now likely to have a cycle lasting perhaps six or seven weeks, with a corresponding reduction in frequency of ovulation and thus in her chances of conceiving. When both ovaries are functioning, they generally alternate in releasing eggs; after a unilateral oophorectomy, the remaining ovary often compensates somewhat. If it's normal, it will react to oral contraceptives as before.

Your patient's questions may reflect a fear that loss of reproductive capacity has diminished her as a woman. You may ease her emotional adjustment to the surgery by encouraging her to express her feelings about it and by assuring her that they're shared by many women who undergo oophorectomy. We'd include her husband in a frank discussion; he, too, is likely to be in conflict over the surgery. To allay concern over the woman's ability to conceive, you might mention that clomiphene (Clomid) and other fertility drugs have helped in just such situations.

* *Can use of oil interfere with conception?*

Can the use of a lubricant such as baby oil interfere with conception if it's rubbed on the penis or female genitalia prior to intercourse? My husband and I enjoy massaging each other during sex play, but now we're trying to have a baby and don't want to do anything that might decrease our chances.

While baby oil and other lubricants aren't reliable contraceptives, they could interfere with fertilization by posing a physical barrier to sperm and altering the chemistry of the vagina. You needn't discontinue your massages, however. Just use the lotion on parts of the body other than the genitals.

* *Impaired fertility from jockey shorts*

I have been having difficulty conceiving and have read that an increase in scrotal temperature causes a decrease in sperm production. Would my chances for conception be improved if my husband switched from jockey shorts to boxer shorts?

Some infertility specialists we know believe so. While the evidence is hardly overwhelming, we feel that in this delicate area it's wise to shade the odds in your favor as much as you can. Therefore, it may well be prudent for your husband to switch to boxer shorts.

* Chances of defects when first cousins marry

A patient is planning to marry her first cousin and wonders how great a chance there is that their children will be abnormal. What shall I tell her?

The answer depends on how many highly deleterious recessive genes each of the couple's common grandparents carried on their autosomes (chromosomes other than those determining sex). This number is unknown, but is estimated to be between two and eight in most people. If there are two, each child of a first-cousin couple would theoretically be at a 1:16 risk of having a recessive disorder.

However, predicting abnormalities in specific consanguineous marriages is enormously complex. For example, parents might have several lines of common ancestry, a frequent phenomenon in small or isolated communities where families often inbreed. Moreover, they may come from an ethnic group or family with a high frequency of specific genetic abnormalities, which would multiply the risk. If one of their children manifests an autosomal recessive abnormality, that establishes that both parents are carriers—and the true risk for each subsequent child then becomes 1:4.

We'd therefore suggest that you put your patient and her cousin in touch with a professional genetic counselor, who can take their family histories and estimate the actual risks. If a counselor isn't affiliated with your hospital, you can probably get a recommendation from the obstetrics or pediatrics department. Or you can query a local chapter of the March of Dimes Birth Defects Foundation or its national headquarters (1275 Mamaroneck Ave., White Plains, N.Y. 10605; telephone 914-428-7100).

* Body temperature and gender determination

Is there any truth to the belief that the sex of the fetus can be influenced by body temperature or season of the year?

We've seen no evidence of it. Because of the body's temperature-regulating mechanisms, the temperature of the reproductive system is generally constant in all climates. Moreover, whether they're carrying X (for female) or Y (for male) chromosomes, sperm cells react to heat and cold in the same way.

* *Effects on sperm movement—and on fetal sex*

Could scheduling intercourse for certain days during the menstrual cycle improve a woman's chances of conceiving a child of a particular sex? Would the woman's position have an influence, since the male-producing sperm swim faster?

No on both counts. You've probably heard speculations that the pH of vaginal secretions changes during the menstrual cycle and that this variation possibly impedes sperm carrying X chromosomes (yielding girls) more than it does sperm carrying Y chromosomes (for boys).

There's been no scientific confirmation of this. The normal pH of the vagina is always acid, and what slight changes occur have not been shown to work for or against either type of sperm.

Similarly, it's a myth that sperm carrying Y chromosomes swim faster than those carrying X chromosomes. Anyway, if male-specifying sperm could swim faster, why would the woman's coital position make any difference? Presumably the Y-carriers would beat out the X-carriers whatever the orientation of the woman's body.

* *Drano: No indicator of fetal sex*

I've heard that if morning urine is added to the drain-cleaning product Drano, the mixture will turn blue if the woman is carrying a boy, brown if a girl. Is this true?

Not in the least. The only way to tell the sex of a fetus is through a chromosome examination of amniotic cells obtained from amniocentesis.

CHAPTER 12

*

Masturbation

*

MASTURBATION IS a nearly universal sexual outlet. Kinsey reported that it is a form of sexual experience shared by 95 percent of the men and 80 percent of the women he surveyed.

But since we live in a society in which many view masturbation as a sin—and in which many believe it has severe physical and emotional consequences as well—it's no surprise that many people experience emotional conflicts over masturbating.

Nor is it surprising if health professionals are in a quandary over how to address masturbation in patients. To deal with the subject sensibly and effectively, the following facts can be helpful.

The exploration of the body and its sexual sensations can be a healthy growth process, leading to enhanced sexual responsiveness. Masturbation has never been proven to impair health or fertility in any way, no matter how often it's engaged in. Physiologically, there's no such thing as excessive masturbation. A person generally stops when it is no longer pleasurable and resumes when it is enjoyable again—all safely and without further consequences.

Contrary to myth, masturbation will not cause acne, warts, hairy palms, gonorrhea, epilepsy, bedwetting, consumption, or blindness. In healthy people, it will not decrease initiative; it will not sidetrack the desire to meet members of the opposite sex.

Hospitalized patients may use masturbation to relieve sexual tension. You might anticipate this need by ensuring them periods of privacy.

* What to do when elderly patients masturbate

I work in a geriatric facility. Several patients, male and female, even in their 90s, masturbate.

One male patient frequently handles his penis and scrotum. His groin is red, and he has required frequent treatments on all shifts. He has an indwelling Foley catheter.

Can he actually have an erection with a catheter present? And would orgasm be as satisfying physically and psychologically?

Several of the nurses are quite disgusted and often rude toward this patient. I have been hesitant about speaking to his doctor.

Yes, erection is possible with a catheter. And yes, so is orgasm with all its physical and psychological satisfactions.

But even more interesting than your questions are the sex-related conflicts you describe between patients and staff. Your report that patients "even in their 90s" masturbate puts the lie to the widespread belief—apparently held by some of your colleagues—that the aging have no sexual needs. Of course they do, as your patients clearly demonstrate.

When geriatric patients masturbate, they're often making use of the only sexual outlet available to them. A compassionate view might be that it's nice they can find at least that much relief. We'd encourage your staff to provide such patients with the privacy that befits any sexual activity.

But this isn't likely to happen as long as nurses are disgusted. What are they disgusted about? Are they made uncomfortable by the act of masturbation? By the fact that it's performed by an elderly patient? Each nurse needs to examine her psychosexual value system to make sure she's not imposing her own prejudices on someone else. A staff conference on geriatric sexuality—and younger persons' attitudes toward it—may prove helpful.

Which brings us to your male patient. By all means, we'd inform his physician of all the problems pertaining to him. But first, we'd be prepared to answer a number of questions.

Why is his groin red? If from handling, a lubricant may be helpful. Perhaps his hands are rough and would benefit from a lotion. More likely, his groin is red because there's a leakage of urine from the Foley. This can often be resolved by keeping the area clean and dry. Is there an infection? Patients with indwelling catheters often suffer from urethritis, and females from vaginitis as well. Their constant handling of their genitals may be an attempt to relieve itching and burning.

How can the patient's relationship with the staff be improved? If your patient is as isolated as he sounds, he may be masturbating to relieve his loneliness—and possibly to get attention, however negative it may be. A deliberate effort to socialize with this patient would seem very much in order.

* *What to say to a masturbating patient*

What would you do if you came across a patient masturbating?

We'd say, "Excuse me. Let me give you some privacy." Then we'd close the door or pull the curtain.

Since even health professionals are affected by taboos regarding masturbation, it can't be repeated too often that the practice is normal, harmless, even beneficial. Besides relieving patient's sexual tensions, around bedtime it can help them relax and fall asleep.

* *Dealing with masturbation as a hostile act*

On the psychiatric unit where I work, I was interviewing a male patient when he suddenly took out his penis and began to masturbate. I interpreted his behavior as an intimidation tactic aimed at terminating the session. In response, I did in fact end the interview, telling him that I would return later that shift when perhaps he'd be more receptive to communication.

I'm not confident that I handled this situation adequately, because I later felt that the patient manipulated me and accomplished his obvious goal of dismissing me. Should I have ignored his hostile, aggressive behavior and continued the interview? Should I have confronted him more directly as to his inappropriate activity? How would you handle such a situation?

For the most part we'd handle the situation much as you did. Apparently, the patient was challenging you for control of the session. It would have been virtually impossible for you to actually ignore his inappropriate behavior. And, if you'd tried to, you'd have been surrendering to his psychopathology. Moreover, since his aim was to resist you, you probably wouldn't have achieved your objectives in the interview anyway; he'd most likely have found ways to thwart you until you left.

To remain in control, you might suspend the interview with a remark like, "I'll return when you're ready to talk." You also might address his masturbation by telling him you'll come back later, when he's finished, and talk about why he decided to do this in front of you. That way, you neutralize his use of masturbation as a tactic and leave the room on your own terms.

* *Masturbation in marriage*

A wife complains that her husband frequently masturbates, often in front of her. He insists that he loves her and that she shouldn't be offended. Is this practice considered normal behavior for a happily married man?

Masturbation, by wives as well as husbands, is part of the sexual activity of a large number of happily married couples. You can assure your patient that her husband's masturbating almost certainly doesn't reflect on his feelings toward her; he may simply enjoy the sensations he derives from masturbating, which can be different and more intense than those from intercourse. In addition, his sexual pleasure is apparently enhanced if he knows that she is observing him, a degree of exhibitionism that's extremely common.

She, of course, has a right not to be an involuntary voyeur, and her preferences, as well as his, must be considered. We've often seen this sort of sexual problem resolved through compromise, especially after the partners recognized that there's nothing necessarily pathological about it. Chances are your patient and her husband can work out an understanding in which each partner respects the other's wishes.

* *Handling a child who masturbates in public*

In the school where I'm a nurse, an 11-year-old girl has been masturbating in class since she was five. I've assured the child and her parents and teachers that masturbation is a normal activity. At the same time, I've told her that, because of other people's sensibilities, she should do it only in private.

I've suggested that her teachers give her an alternative physical activity (running an errand, washing the chalkboard) when they notice her masturbating. I had hoped that with maturation she'd at last stop doing it in public. Now, however, it's come to a crisis: She has male teachers who find her activity extremely disconcerting.

Medical examinations have ruled out vaginitis and other conditions that could cause genital itching. The school physician and psychologist and her family doctor are at a loss. Despite my counseling, her mother considers masturbation to be sinful. She resists psychological counseling for the child, because she feels that would amount to admitting that her daughter is mentally ill. What do you suggest?

Tell the parents that it's crucial for the girl to have a consultation with a child psychiatrist if she is to remain in class. They must be made aware that her behavior is not only pathological but also unacceptable. They wouldn't permit her to, say, urinate in public. There's no reason for them to expect your school to permit exposure of children and teachers to any similar sort of disturbance.

The child may be demonstrating the relatively rare syndrome of compulsive masturbation, not to be confused with ordinary masturbation, which is nearly universal. Like other compulsive acts, this robotlike masturbating occurs with great frequency, continues over long periods, and takes the child's attention away from friends, school, and family. It's mechanical, driven, and essentially joyless; it doesn't seem to offer the child relief, sexual or otherwise.

Compulsive masturbation is but one sign of chronic anxiety. Hostility is another emotion often underlying persistent masturbation in public or in plain view of family members or school authorities. The more open and provocative the masturbating, the more likely that it's being used as a weapon. The only way to stop such behavior humanely is to relieve the emotional conflicts that are causing it.

You and your colleagues are to be congratualted for your sympathetic, enlightened attitude. Usually it's sufficient to explain to a boy or girl, as you did, that masturbating is all right, but the sort of thing people do behind closed doors. It's also wise, as you indicate, to check whether a child's constant genital touching results from pinworms, skin irritations, ill-fitting clothing, phimosis in boys, clitoral adhesions in girls, or other similar causes. When such measures don't work, as in this case, public masturbation is generally a symptom of emotional stress.

* Possible dangers from vibrators

A patient fears that her miscarriage was caused by overuse of a vibrator on her genitals. Can a vibrator cause faulty implantation or make the fetus break away from the uterine wall? Are there other problems associated with vibrators?

You can assure your patient that miscarriages usually result from abnormal germ tissue. Implantation is in no way influenced by the use of a vibrator before or during pregnancy. Nor can the orgasm resulting from this localized tingling cause the fetus to "break away."

Your patient may be feeling guilty about using a vibrator, possibly in masturbation. We'd reassure her that it generally gives pleasure without harm and that its use is widespread and medically permissible.

Offer patients a few caveats, however: A vibrator *can* bruise, tear, and inflame delicate tissues. Before being inserted, it should be lubricated, then introduced slowly. If it becomes at all uncomfortable, it should be removed. While it's inside, a sex partner's weight shouldn't press on it.

Before going from the anus into the vagina, the vibrator should be cleaned. Otherwise, it can carry rectal bacteria and parasities.

It's possible to have an allergic reaction to a vibrator's plastic, rubber, or metal parts. Your patients should be especially wary if they've suffered contact dermatitis elsewhere on the body, as from nickel jewelry or rubber gloves. Use of the device should be stopped at the first sign of reddening, swelling, itching, or blistering. Allergic women may have a vaginal discharge.

Warm-water baths and douches may relieve the inflammation. If not, an estrogen cream (dienestrol or Premarin) may be prescribed to promote vaginal healing. Persistent irritation requires an internal exam.

CHAPTER 13

*

Homosexuality

*

INCREASINGLY, HOMOSEXUALITY is being understood as a basic condition of life for some people, a phenomenon like left-handedness or blue eyes, which just *is* without necessarily having a pathological cause. The American Psychiatric Association no longer considers homosexuality as an illness; similarly, the American Medical Association no longer considers it a disease syndrome.

Homosexuals are thought to constitute about 4 percent of the adult male population and about 2 percent of the adult female population.

As a group, sexually active homosexual males suffer a relatively high rate of venereal disease. A homosexual couple in an exclusive relationship generally have little risk of contracting sexually transmitted diseases, whereas those who have many different partners are at particularly high risk for gonorrhea, nongonococcal urethritis, syphilis, hepatitis, and genital herpes.

These venereal diseases often go unnoticed, or are misdiagnosed. They may be in the throat and rectum and are frequently asymptomatic. Men who have oral or anal sex with many partners are advised to have cultures of the pharynx, urethra, and rectum taken every three to six months in order to detect gonorrhea. Homosexuals with many sexual contacts should consider being vaccinated against hepatitis B. The new vaccine (Heptavax-B) is thought to give protection for up to five years.

Other infections common among homosexuals include such intestinal infections as giardiasis, amebiasis, salmonellosis, and shigellosis. The mode of transmission is usually oral-anal contact or anal intercourse followed by oral sex.

Anal intercourse may result in rectal injury. Venereal warts and pubic lice are also frequently seen among homosexuals.

Homosexuals with many sex partners are at risk for acquired immune deficiency syndrome (AIDS)—a blanket term for several conditions that may result from impaired immunity. One of these conditions is pneumocystosis, an interstitial plasma cell pneumonia with virtually a 100 percent mortality rate in untreated patients.

AIDS often terminates in Kaposi's sarcoma (multiple idiopathic hemorrhagic sarcoma), which begins as soft, brownish or purple papules on the feet and slowly spreads in the skin, metastasizing to the lymph nodes and viscera. Be on the lookout for these suggestive signs of AIDS in your homosexual patients:

- Enlarged lymph nodes in the neck, armpits, or groin. They may be painless.
- Painless purple papules or nodules on the body or inside the mouth, nose, or anus. They may look like bruises, and are usually small at first but may enlarge gradually.
- Unexplained loss of weight.
- Unexplained fever.
- Night sweats for several weeks.
- Dry, hacking cough not associated with a cold.
- Persistent unexplained diarrhea.

* *What to do when a gay patient's lover comes to visit*

One of my postcoronary patients is a male homosexual whose demonstrative visits with his lover upset the other patients. What do you advise?

Ideally, you'd be able to rearrange rooms so that the gay patient is in with roommates who aren't disturbed by his relationship. But even if you can't do that, it's important to protect his emotional lifeline, giving his partner the same consideration you would a heterosexual spouse. This includes extended visiting hours, consultations with staff, and so on.

How can you assure this without causing the other patients uncalled-for annoyance? The best strategy we've seen was the one adopted by a head nurse we'll call Carla. In just such a situation, she told the gay patient: "I feel it's very important for you to have your lover's support. He's as welcome as a close family member, and I'm pleased to work with him for your recovery.

"But," Carla continued, "some of the other patients feel threatened when you show your affection, and I have to consider their well-being as well as yours. So please make everybody more comfortable by closing the curtain or walking to the solarium when you want to be alone."

* Vaginal exams by a lesbian nurse

I am an RN and a lesbian. My sexual orientation isn't obvious to patients and hasn't caused problems with my colleagues, until now.

A new RN on the floor has learned I'm gay. One day, she questioned whether I should be allowed to perform a manual vaginal exam on one of my patients. To avoid any conflict, I immediately asked another nurse to assist me with the exam.

I assure you that I find nothing sexually arousing about examining a vagina—or about performing any other procedures, such as catheterization, involving the female genitalia.

Nevertheless, should I have another nurse assist me with such procedures, as a male physician would have a female nurse present at gynecological exams? I'm afraid this would only draw attention to my sexual preference and cause me to lose my job.

We see no need for such assistance. If a nurse is performing her professional duties satisfactorily, her private preferences are irrelevant—whether sexual, political, or religious.

The problem seems to lie not with your care of patients but with your new colleague's hostile attitude. She apparently feels very threatened by homosexuality. We'd suggest that you sit down with her and quietly and calmly address her fears.

What does she imagine lesbians are like? She might believe that homosexuality is a mental disorder. The American Psychiatric Association has explicitly rejected this view, in part because personality and family studies have been unable to find any significant differences between so-called gays and straights. A more realistic view is that sexual orientation is simply one of many possible variations among human beings, determined in a given individual by biological, psychodynamic, sociocultural, and situational factors too numerous to count.

Your colleague's revulsion toward homosexuality may also be rooted in moral convictions derived from religious beliefs. Here we're dealing with value systems, and she'll have to recognize that not everyone may share her view of right and wrong. A nurse is free to adhere to her personal moral code in the conduct of her private life. In the performance of her professional duties, however, she must be extremely careful not to impose her morality on others.

You might assure your colleague that you obey the same professional taboos as she does against getting sexually involved with patients. People who fancy that homosexuals are mentally ill often don't realize that gay persons have the same behavior controls as anyone else. You can tell her that you're as unlikely to take advantage of a female patient as she is to take advantage of a male patient. Further, you might reassure her that there's no possibility you'll make a pass at her, a common fear of heterosexuals who are unfamiliar with gay people's behavior.

Unfortunately, you're on the defensive in this situation. However, confronting your colleague in a warm and honest fashion may defuse her hostility and help her realize that the label lesbian has prevented her from seeing you as a person and professional.

But what if you fail? What if she continues to harass you? Then you have grounds to complain to your supervisor, who should treat the situation just as she would any conflict caused by one nurse's unwarranted hostility toward another.

* Same-sex play: Is it homosexuality?

On returning home from a party unexpectedly early, a patient and her husband found their 15-year-old son naked in bed with another boy, engaging in mutual masturbation. The parents reacted rather abusively. How do you suggest such situations be handled? Does this mean the boy is or will become a homosexual?

Any time parents come upon their children engaging in sexual activity with a friend—whether of the same or other sex—it's a good idea to say something like, "Let me give you kids a chance to get yourselves together." This gives all parties a breather. When everyone's calmed down, you might tell the youngsters that walking in on such a scene makes you very uncomfortable and that they should take care it doesn't happen again.

Without evidence to the contrary, it's probable that the boy in this case is going through a stage of psychosexual development that's widespread but little-discussed. It's extremely common for boys and girls to engage in sexual experimentation with members of their own sex. Adolescents are often in a state of high sexual tension that can be discharged with either sex. A member of the other sex may not be available. And, even if one were accessible, sexual involvement might well be premature in the youngster's overall development.

Thus, among adolescents, an incident such as you've described is usually homosexual only in the sense that it occurs within the same gender. It rarely indicates homosexuality, a basic sexual and emotional affinity toward one's own sex.

CHAPTER 14

*

Drugs and Sex

*

IN DETERMINING the causes of sexual dysfunctions, it's important to keep in your differential any chemicals your patients are taking into their bodies. Sex can be affected in some degree by most drugs, including prescription and nonprescription medications as well as social or recreational drugs such as alcohol, tobacco, and marijuana.

As causative factors in sexual dysfunction, the effects of drugs may be subtle. Their sexual side effects vary greatly from person to person. The precise reaction depends on absorption rate, body weight, rate of metabolism, length of use, excretion rate, dosage, interactions with other drugs, and other variables.

Because the potential for sexual side effects of drugs isn't widely appreciated, your patients may be alarmed by unexplained sexual dysfunctions. Thus, it's a good idea to caution patients about the possible sexual consequences of the drugs they take.

* *Impotence and cimetidine*

A duodenal ulcer patient complains of impotence since starting to take cimetidine (Tagamet). Is there a connection?

Could be. The drug may act as an antiandrogen. It has been associated with impotence, loss of sexual desire, and low sperm counts. Your patient might try discontinuing the drug under a physician's supervision, to see if his erectile capacity returns.

* *Can bromocriptine help a woman achieve orgasm?*

I've heard that bromocriptine mesylate (Parlodel) can help previously anorgasmic women reach orgasm. Is this true?

So it seems. The drug is usually used to suppress lactation after delivery and also to treat amenorrhea and galactorrhea associated with hyperprolactinemia. It acts like testosterone and evidently gives some women a feeling of well-being that promotes their sexual arousal.

However, bromocriptine is no substitute for relaxation and pleasuring as a means of facilitating orgasm. The drug has a high incidence of adverse reactions and should never be used for more than six months. In addition, its antiestrogen effect counteracts oral contraceptives, so another form of birth control is necessary during treatment. And bromocriptine may lead to early postpartum conception; a pregnancy test is required every four months or, after menses are reinitiated, whenever the patient misses a period.

* *How steroids may affect sex*

Do steroids have sexual side effects?

Short-term use of corticosteroids, over a course of up to 10 days, seems to have no adverse effect on a patient's sexual function. However, long-term use has a number of side effects that can result in a loss of sexual desire—an early warning sign your patients should know about.

Long-term use of steroids is, for instance, often related to depression and other mental disturbances that may impair sexual function. More directly, steroids over a long term may suppress secretion of sex hormones by interfering with the output of pituitary gonadotropin.

The drugs may further have an impact on your patient's sexual functioning by causing muscle weakness, vertigo, and headache. Steroids can produce hyperglycemia and can precipitate latent diabetes, with accompanying impotence. They may sometimes alter your patient's appearance, causing moon face, hirsutism, and excess fat.

Your male patients may become infertile while on steroids—large doses (30 mg/day of prednisone) have been observed to depress production of sperm. Women may suffer amenorrhea or menstrual irregularity. Steroids also put women at increased risk of vaginal infection. Prolonged use of steroids, including steroid creams under occlusive dressings, may produce stretch marks.

Paradoxically, long-term use of steroids can also cause your patient to feel euphoric; consequent relief of depression and anxiety can enhance sexual activity.

* *Barbiturates and sexual function*

Several patients who take sleeping pills complain that they've lost their desire for sex. Is there a connection?

There could be. At the beginning of therapy, barbiturates sometimes reduce sexual inhibitions, enhancing sexual enjoyment. But, for both men and women, chronic use often results in a decrease in libido and difficulty in attaining orgasm. In addition, men may become impotent and women may experience menstrual abnormalities.

* *Sexual side effects of diuretics*

A male patient taking a diuretic for congestive heart failure is experiencing breast enlargement with tenderness and pain. Could the drug be the cause?

Very possibly, if he's taking spironolactone alone (Aldactone) or in combination with hydrochlorothiazide (Aldactazide). Spironolactone evidently affects the endocrine system and can cause gynecomastia and mastodynia. This drug can also cause impotence, loss or decrease of libido, menstrual irregularities, and inhibition of vaginal lubrication. Thiazide and related diuretics infrequently impair libido and vaginal lubrication and occasionally cause impotence. Having his physician switch him to another medication may reduce your patient's adverse reactions.

* *Possible adverse effects of allergy medications*

My husband is allergic to just about everything. For the past four years he has been receiving two allergy shots a month. He's also been taking antihistamines daily; his current medication is a PBZ-with-ephedrine combination. Can sexual dysfunction result from such therapy? Is there any danger of impotence or birth defects?

Antihistamines often have a sedative effect that can depress libido. In men, this may lead to impotence; in women, antihistamines can impair vaginal lubrication.

If your husband does experience impotence, it may be due to the antihistamine tripelennamine, the PBZ part of his prescription. Such adverse sexual effects might be reduced by holding off the drug until after having intercourse. A modified dosage or a switch to another product could also prove helpful.

For women who experience a decrease in vaginal lubrication due to antihistamines, the use of contraceptive jelly or a water-soluble lubricant is advisable.

The safety of antihistamines during pregnancy and lactation hasn't been established, so the drugs shouldn't be used by women who are pregnant or nursing. There's no evidence that birth defects can result from ordinary use of antihistamines, however, nor have we seen any adverse sexual effects or teratogenic effects from ephedrine or from allergenic extracts used for diagnosis or immunotherapy.

* *Phenothiazines: Their effect on sex*

A patient taking thioridazine (Mellaril) for schizophrenia complains of painful ejaculation. To what extent might this be due to the drug? To the schizophrenia? To his masturbating? What sexual side effects are associated with phenothiazines?

Neither schizophrenia nor masturbation ordinarily causes ejaculatory pain. However, it is one of the most frequent male sexual dysfunctions associated with thioridazine. Painful ejaculation, retrograde ejaculation, absent or markedly reduced ejaculate at orgasm, and impotence are other frequent side effects. Women taking thioridazine may experience amenorrhea and delayed ovulation.

Phenothiazines as a class produce a sedative effect that can diminish sexual desire; such loss of libido is most widely reported with chlorpromazine (Thorazine). In addition, many phenothiazines have potent anticholinergic effects that may produce vaginal dryness, impotence, or ejaculatory difficulties, especially at doses equivalent to 400 mg/day or more of chlorpromazine. The drugs also can block ovulation, cause menstrual irregularities, induce galactorrhea or gynecomastia, and decrease testicular size. Further, phenothiazines potentiate alcohol, barbiturates, and narcotics, intensifying such sexual side effects as impotence and reduced libido.

* *Does saltpeter lower the sex drive?*

It's long been rumored that saltpeter lowers the male sex drive and so is added to food at boarding schools, prisons, and military camps. Does saltpeter actually have such an effect?

No. Saltpeter (potassium nitrate or sodium nitrate) is used as a meat preservative and has a mild diuretic action, but no effects on sexual interest or capacity. In all-male settings, it's not uncommon for a man to find he has fewer erections than usual. That's probably because the environment provides little sexual stimulation and may be depressing.

In the 18th and 19th centuries, saltpeter was used to bring down fevers because it was erroneously thought to cool the body. Since folklore associates sexual excitement with heat, the myth of saltpeter as an anaphrodisiac may have sprung from this supposed effect.

No responsible institution would add saltpeter to its food to quell the sex drive. To do so would risk poisoning the diners. In toxic quantities, saltpeter causes vomiting, severe gastrointestinal pain, and profuse purgation. Prompt emesis is required.

* *Dangerous effects of Spanish fly*

I've heard a great deal of talk about Spanish fly as an aphrodisiac. What is it? Does it work?

Spanish fly is the popular name for cantharidin, a product of *Lytta (Cantharis) vesicatoria*, a beetle found in southern Europe. From Greek and Roman times to the early part of this century, the substance was widely ingested as a sexual stimulant and administered surreptitiously to promote seductions.

Actually it's an extremely irritating chemical that enters the urine and inflames the ureters, bladder, and urethra. This inflammation may cause an unsettled sensation in the genital region and possibly an erection.

Cantharidin is such a strong vesicant, however, that its only medical use is as a wart remover. Probably more people have been injured or killed by the chemical than have been sexually stimulated by it. Poisoning by cantharidin leads to abdominal pain and frequent painful passage of urine, often containing blood and sloughed bladder mucosa. There may be blisters along the urethra and on the end of the penis. The only antidote is the administration of large volumes of fluids to dilute the poison in the urine.

* *Effects of amyl nitrite poppers*

Some of my patients say they intensify their orgasms by popping an amyl nitrite vial and inhaling the vapor. Can you explain the sexual effects of this drug? Is the practice harmful?

Amyl nitrite is a fast-acting smooth-muscle relaxant and coronary vasodilator, originally used to relieve attacks of angina pectoris. The drug probably causes engorgement of the genitourinary vessels, which could cause a heightened rush during the decongestion accompanying orgasm. By abruptly lowering blood pressure, the drug also may produce feelings of dizziness and giddiness that add to the experience. Cutaneous vasodilation may make the skin more sensitive, enhancing the pleasure of tactile stimulation.

We've seen no reports of serious complications among users of poppers, as the amyl nitrite vials are popularly known. Nonetheless, it's prudent to warn against their recreational use by patients with cardiovascular or cerebrovascular disease. Hypotension, tachycardia, and a small increase followed by a reduction in cardiac output may pose dangers to these individuals. The drug may also transiently raise intraocular pressure, making its safety for patients with glaucoma and other ocular diseases questionable.

You can tell your patients that the most common side effect is a typical severe nitrite headache from dilation of blood vessels in the extracranial circulation. This discomfort is usually short-lived and rarely dangerous.

Also, caution your patients that they risk fainting, especially if they drink alcohol, which has an additive hypotensive effect. A final precaution: Amyl nitrite vapors are highly flammable, so shouldn't be used near a flame or intense heat that could cause them to ignite.

A related chemical, butyl nitrite, is widely sold in head shops, ostensibly as a room deodorizer. Its chief use is actually as a recreational drug. You can warn patients that it has essentially the same side effects as amyl nitrite.

* Alcohol-induced impotence

How does alcohol affect erections? As head nurse of an alcoholic detox and rehab unit, I've heard many patients complain of impotence. What's their prognosis with abstinence from alcohol?

As Shakespeare had Macbeth's porter observe of drink, "It provokes the desire, but takes away the performance." Alcohol evidently depresses the pudendal nerves and erection reflex; it is the second most common cause of impotence (after physical or emotional fatigue). That "one drink too many" explains why couples coming home from a party are often disappointed when they try to make love.

The effect depends on the individual's tolerance to alcohol and may be subtle. We've seen many a man who has a martini for lunch and another after work, wine with dinner, then a cognac with his coffee. He doesn't feel drunk or even think of himself as drinking, but his blood alcohol level may be high enough to prevent an erection. His tolerance may be even lower if he smokes, is under stress, doesn't watch his diet, or suffers from poor health.

In advanced alcoholism, patients often suffer from neuropathy and liver problems, both of which can cause organic impotence. The improvement of the sexual dysfunction depends on how well the tissues repair. Thus, when your patients stop drinking, it's a good idea to be conservative with your sexual prognosis.

We tell recovering alcoholics that their organic impotence is likely to take at least three months to improve. Meanwhile, to forestall psychogenic impotence, we encourage them to engage in intimate activity without expectation of intercourse. Recovering alcoholics often demonstrate the interplay between organic and psychogenic impotence. A man whose impotence is supposedly due to physiological damage may benefit from sexual counseling.

* *Smoking and impotence*

A college student in his 20s complains that he's frequently unable to get or sustain an erection. His health picture is unremarkable, except that he smokes two packs of cigarettes a day. Could this contribute to his erectile dysfunction?

It certainly could. Smoking even less than two packs a day can have, in some men, enough of a vasoconstrictive effect to reduce the penile blood supply needed for an erection. His smoking can also impair his pulmonary function, promoting fatigue and loss of erection during active intercourse. Moreover, his smoking may leave odors on his breath and body that his partners find unpleasant; their withdrawal from him is likely to decrease his sexual arousal, even though neither partner is consciously aware of the rejection.

* *Smoking as a fetish*

My husband smokes only when he's engaging in sex play. He also finds it sexually stimulating to watch me or other women smoke. I don't like tobacco, but I smoke to please him, averaging about 10 cigarettes a month. Will this harm my health? How can smoking be a stimulant? Does my husband suffer from a fetish?

Any smoking assaults the tissues and ideally should be avoided. Statistically, however, smoking a mere one cigarette every three days or so is likely to have only a negligible long-term effect on your health. Without impinging on your husband's pleasure, you can reduce the risks to yourself by not inhaling.

Your husband's sexual response is probably enhanced by the acute effect of nicotine, which stimulates sensory receptors and increases the heart rate and blood pressure. His reaction to females smoking could be said to constitute fetishism, which is the arousal of erotic feelings by an action, object, or body part that's not primarily sexual in nature.

Contrary to popular belief, a fetish doesn't necessarily indicate psychopathology. Often, as seems to be the case in your marriage, it's incorporated into an otherwise satisfying sexual relationship. As long as no one is truly suffering, there's little reason to alter the behavior.

CHAPTER 15

*

Sexual Dysfunction

*

IT'S ESTIMATED that half of all marriages suffer from some degree of sexual dysfunction. The most common sex disorders are impotence, premature ejaculation, orgasmic problems, and diminished sexual desire.

Before referring patients for psychological counseling or sex therapy, rule out organic problems. For many patients, sexual orders are the result of illness, medications, surgery, or congenital malformations of the urogenital system.

Myths about sex frequently contribute to sexual dysfunction. In our experience, one out of four people experiencing sexual difficulties can be cured by simple reassurance and education about their bodies.

Urge your patients to think of sexual activity not as a contact sport with orgasm as the goal but rather as a pleasurable continuum of shared experiences. Remind them that there is much more to sex than a penis inside a vagina. Indeed, a couple can have a mutually satisfying sexual experience without penetration or orgasm.

* *Etiology of painful intercourse*

A women reports finding intercourse painful, even though she's adequately stimulated prior to intromission and thus can't ascribe her discomfort to lack of lubrication. Can you suggest what's causing her problem?

We'd first rule out organic causes, especially vaginal infection or inflammation. We'd then determine when and where the pain occurs.

Dyspareunia deep in the vagina may be due to pelvic inflammatory disease, endometriosis, uterine fibroids, or surgical adhesions.

If the pain is at the vaginal opening, it may result from a hymenal residue or a scar. Introital pain can also arise from such postdelivery trauma as episiotomy, generally with suture granuloma formation. When a scar is the cause of dyspareunia, it's usually painful when stretched digitally. The problem can be corrected by surgery.

As you suggest, lack of lubrication is the most frequent cause of coital pain, and such inadequate arousal typically is psychogenic and may be resolved with counseling. Even when the cause is primarily organic, there's usually a strong psychological component. After delivery or other severe perineal disturbance, a woman may develop vaginismus (involuntary spasm) from fear of penetration.

In our postoperative counseling, we tell the patient that she may pull back from anticipation of pain. To help her overcome this anxiety, we suggest that she go along with the initial discomfort but concentrate on the pleasures the sex play affords. This often enables her to focus on immediate, enjoyable sensations rather than on her anxiety over what will happen next.

Vaginismus also can be a long-lasting sequel to rape or incest. For such patients, we'd recommend a psychiatric referral.

* *Failure to ejaculate*

I've heard teenagers complain of "blue balls" and older men say they often can't "come" during intercourse. What causes these responses? Is it physically harmful not to ejaculate after arousal?

You can tell older men that, after 40 or so, it's normal to occasionally feel no physical need to ejaculate. A man may be fully potent and enjoy all other aspects of coitus. He'll reach the plateau stage, and then his erection will subside without orgasm. The next time, he probably will ejaculate.

"Blue balls" is a form of epididymo-orchitis. Vasocongestion leading to testicular ache results from ungratified sexual excitement, often petting without ejaculatory relief.

Teenagers are especially susceptible to it because of their dating patterns and because they're at a stage of heightened physical responsiveness. Some boys fear they'll suffer permanent damage—and some may tell their girlfriends that in an attempt to pressure them into intercourse. In fact, the condition is self-limiting: All the boy need do is go home and masturbate.

Repeated episodes of sexual arousal without ejaculation may lead to congestive prostatitis (also called prostatosis or pelvic congestion syndrome). It's marked by perineal ache, low back pain, pelvic and suprapubic pressure, and frequent painful urination. There may be a clear urethral discharge and bloody ejaculation. Rectal examination reveals a tense, tender prostate. If prolonged, prostatosis may produce partial obstruction of the bladder and bacterial prostatitis.

The condition often affects men who go through feast-or-famine sexual cycles: The prostate increases its secretion of prostatic fluid to meet higher demands, then becomes congested on sudden cessation of sexual activity. We also know of one man who developed the pelvic congestion syndrome as a result of his job as a proofreader in a pornographic publishing house. He was awarded workers' compensation.

At the beginning of treatment, it's necessary to rule out bacterial infection, which has many of the same symptoms as the congestive condition. When the problem *is* an infection, however, there are bacteria and pus cells in the expressed prostatic secretion; acute bacterial prostatitis is further characterized by the sudden onset of chills and fever, and by general malaise. Semen cultures or fractionated urine cultures can point to the proper antibiotic when these symptoms are present.

What's the treatment for congestive prostatitis? Ejaculation—by any form of sexual activity acceptable to the patient—provides the best means of emptying the seminal vesicles and relieving prostatic congestion. Prostatic massage is a poor and needlessly expensive substitute.

If your patient has no sex partner available, you may need to counsel him on the normalcy and health benefits of masturbation as a way to relieve sexual tension. Many men feel guilty about masturbating, erroneously believing that "it's a habit I should have outgrown." Additional relief may be provided by sitz baths and by such time-honored remedies as the avoidance of alcohol, coffee, and spicy foods.

* *Too old for sex*

A patient's husband, who's 60, suddenly has lost interest in having intercourse and no longer gets erections. He speculates that he's "gotten too old for sex." Is this possible? He doesn't seem depressed or ill and isn't taking any drugs. What do you advise?

You can assure your patient that no age is "too old" for sex, let alone 60. We'd urge that he get a physical exam that includes an oral glucose tolerance test. Impotence can be a prodromal symptom of diabetes, appearing before the classic symptoms of itching, weight loss, polyphagia, polydipsia, and polyuria. In such cases, the impotence typically has rapid onset and is marked by loss of sex drive. It can usually be reversed with good control of the underlying hyperglycemia.

You're perceptive in including depression as a possible cause of impotence. However, psychogenic impotence is rarely marked by complete erectile dysfunction; in such a case. erections generally occur during sleep.

* *How to arouse an older man*

A 70-year-old man, otherwise in good health, has difficulty getting an erection. His wife asks what parts of his body she might best massage to sexually arouse him. What should I tell her?

You can tell her that she's on the right track in regarding lovemaking as a whole-body process and being prepared to stimulate her partner in nongenital ways. The skin virtually everywhere on the body has a highly erogenous potential, and partners can arouse both themselves and each other by massaging, stroking, kissing, and caressing a wide range of sites. After using this approach, a couple we were seeing for sex therapy reported, "We've each discovered ten new sex organs. Our toes!"

You might also tell your patient that, with aging, men often take longer to achieve erections, and those erections may be less firm or long-lasting. Therefore, in addition to the pleasures of whole-body arousal, older men may need direct stimulation of the penis.

* *A wandering mind during sex*

An executive complains that his mind wanders when he's engaging in sex. Physically he's in bed with his wife, but mentally he's dealing with business problems. What can I advise him?

To help him stay in the here and now, you might recommend that he focus on his wife—giving her pleasure and experiencing her reaction. Suggest that he leave a light on—and his eyes open—when making love; otherwise, his mental screen is likely to flood with images born of his business tensions. As soon as he detects his mind drifting, he might restore his concentration by whispering to his wife ("I love you" is always a nice thing to say) and altering his activity.

This executive probably has difficulty relaxing in general and feels guilty about playing. When he's not working, he most likely feels he's wasting his time—and this compulsiveness extends to his sex life.

We've seen many couples whose sex lives have suffered because one or both partners can't let go of a task orientation. Alas, when sex gets low priority in the press of other work, it tends to become a chore itself, a ritual rather than a pleasure.

In our observation, a satisfying sex life requires an ability to take time out. You may need to advise a couple to take the phone off the hook for a couple of hours to give themselves time to relax and enjoy each other.

CHAPTER 16

*

Problems in the Hospital

*

WHEN WORKING in a hospital or nursing home, you may need to deal with such common, but little discussed, sexual issues as these:

- What degree of sexual privacy ought patients have?
- How should you deal with attraction to a patient?
- What do you do if a patient makes sexual advances?
- How should you react when a patient exposes himself?

The following questions discuss these and a variety of other sex-related issues that you may encounter in an institutional setting.

* *Sexual needs of hospitalized patients*

How do you deal with the desire of long-term patients to have intercourse while in the hospital?

Let's not talk about intercourse only, which your question implies is necessarily the goal. The issue is really the larger one of resolving the sexual needs of chronic patients. Indeed, because of illness or its therapy, a patient may not be interested in coitus, yet may crave holding and caressing, the pleasure of stimulating the partner, or other forms of contact.

Not only do chronic patients continue to have sexual needs, the satisfaction of which is good for their emotional and physical condition, but also they are often concerned that their partners won't have sexual release. Respecting your patients as sexually independent adults can help keep them from falling into apathetic, frustrated, destructive "sick patient" roles.

We try to make provision for our patients' sexual expression by securing privacy for them and their partners. We help ambulatory patients who have roommates to borrow an empty room "for a private visit." And we assure bedridden patients that drawn curtains will be as honored as a "Do Not Disturb" sign on the door. This guarantee gives them an opportunity to release sexual tension and fulfill their need for intimate contact—despite the seemingly flimsy barrier that the curtains provide.

* *Providing patients with sexual privacy*

I realize that patients often have unmet sexual needs, especially those in wards or semiprivate rooms who are unable to have time alone with their partners. How can I help change hospital policy to remedy this? What's the best way to raise the subject with patients?

There is a tendency among hospitals to make private rooms available for such visits, and that might be your goal. To achieve it, we'd suggest you get together with like-minded colleagues and speak out at staff meetings in favor of such a provision.

You can expect resistance, however; and it may be necessary to have workshops led by consultants who are oriented toward sexual medicine, focusing not only on the patients' needs but also on the staff members' feelings.

For starters, you might secure sexual privacy for patients in semiprivate rooms while the other patient is gone for a defined period. If your hospital makes provisions such as private rooms, you can approach patients with a statement like, "Would you care to spend a couple of hours alone with your wife? I can arrange for you not to be disturbed."

* *Rules for adolescent patients*

Our pediatric ward has a special wing for patients 12 to 17 years old. We've often found ambulatory youngsters in bed with each other, engaging in sexual activity. How can our staff cope with adolescent social and sexual needs, without coming across like harsh, demanding Puritans?

First of all, we'd schedule daily supervised sessions in which these teenagers can share their feelings about being sick. Patients this age need a lot of support. Much of their sexual activity may result from their striving for warmth, contact, and reassurance.

Thus it's helpful to give them a constructive way to deal with an overwhelming experience. What do their illnesses mean to them? How do they feel about being separated from home, family, and friends? What are their fears about medication, surgery, disfigurement, reduced physical abilities? How much is death on their minds? What do they dislike about hospital life, and how can it be changed?

Encourage group activities. Have the patients eat together. Assign them jobs in twos and threes. As much as possible, give them the opportunity to act like brothers and sisters—talking, arguing, voting. The less alone they feel during this crisis, the less likely they are to seize on sex to break their isolation.

In addition, we'd give them a clear set of rules. The most basic one would be: "Visiting allowed only with the door open." In your discussion groups, spell it out: "No genital sex." You might also work in a good deal of sex education. Put sex in the context of the many ways people express their need for closeness. In this age group, some handholding, touching, and kissing are inevitable—but your patients need not go beyond that.

Indeed, much as we admire your staff's wish to provide a friendly setting for this difficult age group, we wouldn't worry about coming across like Puritans. The first responsibility of health professionals is the welfare of the patient, not being "with it." Your young patients are in a strange environment and may be impaired by illness and medication. Those who've led sheltered lives are thrown in with a rougher bunch. Younger kids are mixed in with older ones.

In our experience, adolescents not only need but also appreciate sexual guidance from health professionals. It's a sign of the pernicious effect of the so-called new morality that you're feeling self-conscious about doing the appropriate thing. Why should it be wrong, in sexual matters as in anything else, to set sensible limits?

You also need such rules for your own protection. In the eyes of the community, you're acting in place of the parent. Your hospital would be in a mighty awkward position—and possibly in legal jeopardy—if a teenager became pregnant while in your care.

* *When a confused patient is molested*

In the nursing home where I work, an alert male patient keeps fondling a female patient who he knows is confused. She is unable to object—or consent—to his actions. What are her rights? How should the situation be handled?

How would you handle *any* situation in which one patient physically assaults another? Patients in your care have an absolute right not to be abused. They also have a right to be protected.

Chances are other patients are aware of the exploitation and fear that they may be vulnerable as well. In the absence of firm, immediate action, your facility is thus threatened with a deterioration in patient morale, a breakdown in interpersonal relationships—and possible lawsuits on behalf of any sexually molested patients.

First of all, we'd tell this man that such behavior is unacceptable if he wishes to remain in the nursing home. To help cool things off, we'd keep him and the woman apart for a few days. Meanwhile, we'd explore with him what he's seeking: Is it attention? Affection? Physical contact? Sexual gratification? Rebellion against authority? You may be able to help him find other ways to satisfy his needs—including a reciprocal relationship with an alert woman.

* How to handle attraction to a patient

I sometimes feel sexual excitement toward young male patients. Aren't such feelings wrong? How can I deal with them?

We'd suggest that you accept these pleasurable stirrings—and have the confidence that they're unlikely to interfere with your professional responsibilities. Far from being "wrong," occasional sexual feelings toward patients seem to be a fact of life for health-care professionals. If this reality were more widely discussed—first in school and then in staff conferences—fewer of us would feel guilty over our involuntary responses.

Your degree in the health sciences has not neutered you, nor are relationships with patients absolutely asexual. If you're like most adults, as you grew up you developed strong positive feelings toward certain traits in your own and the other sex. This imprinting has stayed with you, and you will continue to respond warmly to particular kinds of looks and mannerisms, whether the person you find them in is a patient or not.

As a health worker, you encounter a great many people. Inevitably, some of them exhibit one or more of the qualities that appeal to you. And when one of these happens to be your patient, the probability of your being aroused increases for at least these two reasons: You're supposed to be a caring human being toward this person and you exercise this care on extremely intimate terms.

Sexual contact with patients is so forbidden that many health professionals are frightened by such arousal. But you're unlikely to act out your fantasies—your behavior controls won't let you—so you generally need to be no more embarrassed about your private feelings than you are about your dreams.

Every health professional has favorite types of patients, people whom they're inclined to care for specially and whose good opinion they want in return. Some of us gravitate toward jolly grandpas; others have a soft spot for junior misses. In practice, the extra warmth sometimes felt toward patients is rarely different from that.

Of course, some patients can stir the deepest parts of your psyche, and you'd do well to withdraw if you're really being caught up by your feelings. For example, you may find yourself becoming preoccupied with the patient or being flirtatious with him or touching him in suggestive ways. A CCU nurse told us of a young man to whom she was strongly attracted. "He had this wonderfully hairy chest," she recalled. "I was turned on and I couldn't view his illness objectively." Recognizing the dangers to the patient and herself, she asked that another nurse handle his case.

* *Fielding patients' passes*

How should I handle male patients who make passes? I'm tired of fending off sexual advances, and I've run out of quick comebacks that don't work anyway.

Hospitalized men, especially postcoronary and postoperative patients, often fear for their sexuality because of their general feelings of dependence and helplessness. They tend to see nurses as safe, strong, caring women who are able to handle life-threatening situations—and who are therefore able to take whatever behavior gets aimed at them.

When a patient makes a pass at you, he's probably testing your reaction to him as a sexual being. He's often badly in need of reassurance and seldom intends to follow through. You need only to acknowledge that he's concerned about his sexual ability, and that he's likely missing his loved ones.

An RN we'll call Florence recently handled an amorous patient in precisely that way. Like many nurses, she had been taught, "Ignore the patient's advances, and, if he persists, admonish him for his inappropriate behavior."

Instead, she transcended her traditional training and dealt with her patient's pass in a gentle, sympathetic manner. When Mr. Dunlap made his move, she simply said, "You must be very lonely being away from your loved ones. I imagine it's hard for them, too."

She went on to voice her discomfort. "Even so, when you put your hands on me, it makes me uncomfortable. I know you need to reach out to someone. That's important to all of us. But right now it's interfering with my work."

When Mr. Dunlap figuratively backed off, Florence then offered this positive solution tp his problem: She asked him if there was anyone she could call for him.

* Dealing with amorous doctors

How can a female health worker protect herself from sexually aggressive male physicians on the hospital's staff? I'm often bothered by doctors who speak salaciously and insist on placing their hands everywhere but in their pockets.

Good for you for bringing up this dark corner of hospital life! No nurse need put up with sexual harassment by a physician. If a doctor speaks suggestively to you, you can simply tell him that his language is offensive to you, that it's a distraction that interferes with your performance, and that you'd hate to have to report him.

Treat pawing the same way. Remind the doctor that you're a person first and a nurse second, and that you have a right to decide who's going to touch your body—and when and how.

Realizing that some of these doctors may be sexually unsatisfied and insecure may help. Among our physician-patients in sex therapy we've frequently seen this pattern: The doctor has the same sexual needs as everyone else, but he's a workaholic. He's rarely home, and when he is, he's tired. He and his wife have drifted apart. Thus there's little of the time and warmth needed for a mature, fulfilling, intimate relationship.

In the hospital, the doctor may be sexually aroused by the nurses with whom he works. He also may be aroused by attractive patients—but these impulses are so forbidden that he channels them toward nurses. He seizes on the power his position gives him, which is reinforced by the folk belief held by some physicians that nurses are dumb little sex objects.

And so, frustrated, seeking sexual recognition, and overcompensating for his inadequacies, he becomes sexually aggressive to nurses. He may actually be seeking a liaison or he may merely be acting out his fantasies, while having no intention of following through. In any event, meeting the doctor's sexual needs is not part of any nurse's duties.

You might remedy the situation by helping the doctor to reflect on his inappropriate behavior. When he makes a salacious remark, for example, you could reply, "I hear what you're saying, but I don't think that's what you really want."

We also suggest that you examine your own behavior, to see if you're inadvertently inviting such approaches. In episodes of this sort, the nurse often is party to a game in which the doctor personifies stereotyped masculine traits and she personifies classical feminine ones. Playing out the traditional roles, he acts heroic, dashing, macho, a stud, while she is warm, passive, demure—and seductive.

Personal postscript: Before we were married we worked in the same hospital. A doctor kept making advances to Dotty, who rebuffed him. He complained to Armando, "That new nurse is a cold number. She thinks I'm a dirty old man." Replied Armando: "Maybe you are."

* *Dealing with an exhibitionist*

An alert male patient needlessly exposes his genitals during nursing procedures. He also feigns helplessness, allowing his gown to fall open. How should I respond?

First, we'd suggest that you request a team conference involving the nurses on your unit, your supervisor, the attending physician, and a social worker. This patient is troubled and he's probably exposing himself to other nurses as well. All the nurses should thus be prepared to confront his provocative behavior, and for this you may benefit from professional support and guidance.

Such a confrontation should be private and tactful, with no hint of reprimand. You might start off by asking him if he's aware that he often shows his genitals and if he knows that this isn't acceptable behavior because it can disturb other people. You can go on to explore his motives by saying something like, "When patients do this, they're usually trying to say something. Are you having a tough time with your hospitalization? How can I help you?"

You may find that he's lonely, anxious, frustrated over his medical condition, worried about his sexuality, or angry at the care he's receiving. Once you know what's bothering him, your team can reconvene and decide the best course of action: Arranging for a visitor, counseling, and so on. Sometimes just talking with the patient can resolve the difficulty. He should be made aware that he has your attention and that you really care about him.

* *When a patient wants more than a back rub*

A woman in her early 50s is admitted to my unit from time to time for ulcers. She seems like a nice lady, but she repeatedly asks us to rub not only her back but also such areas as her abdomen and chest. Even though this makes all the staff members uncomfortable, some of the younger ones think they have to "do what the patient wants." This woman also claims she cannot reach her "privates" and asks to be washed there when she showers.

I've told the patient, "We're allowed to rub only your back, and that's that." I've also said to the younger nurses "The good Lord made people's arms long enough to reach down there, and the patient should do this herself." How can we handle this problem better?

We suggest frankly telling the patient that her demands are making the nurses uncomfortable. You could ask her how she manages to wash herself when she's not in the hospital and suggest that she follow the same procedure. Remind her, too, that, unlike some patients, she's lucky enough to be able to take care of herself.

Why is she making such demands? Hospitalization might be making her feel vulnerable and dependent; perhaps she's longing to be treated like a little girl whose loving mother rubs her belly and washes her "privates." She also might generally have difficulty relating to adults, and so may use a childish ploy to gain reassurance that she's cared for. It's also possible that there's a sexual component in the situation; she might be sexually aroused by nurses, and stimulated by their attentions.

On the other hand, your patient might just be lonely. We'd suggest finding out if there's anyone she'd like you to call for her.

* *Enema-induced erection*

When a patient experiences an erection during an enema, does this indicate he's sexually aroused? Or is the erection a reflex action triggered by the pressure of the fluid?

Either or both. The stimulation of the prostate can cause a reflex erection. Enemas can also be sexually arousing and generate erotic fantasies. An impersonal explanation such as the foregoing may help relieve any embarrassment on the part of both you and the patient.

* *When there's an erection during a prep*

While I was prepping a young man for surgery, he experienced an erection. Although I wasn't perturbed, he was extremely embarrassed. I treated the event matter-of-factly and tried to distract him with conversation. Nevertheless, his erection persisted throughout the entire prep.

Now I'm wondering if there was something I could have done to help prevent or stop his erection.

You might have had the patient empty his bladder before the prep, especially if it was early in the day. If he hadn't voided since awakening, he may have had a "morning erection," stimulated by the presence of urine. Aside from this, there's no method we can recommend that would reduce or prevent an erection.

You could have eased his embarrassment by explaining the erection; trying to ignore it or making small talk may have made the patient more tense. You might have told him that his erection was simply the spontaneous result of tactile stimulation and that this response reflects a healthy, intact neuromuscular system.

To do a prep with minimal embarrassment in such a circumstance, drape a towel over the erection and move the penis if it's in your way. Even if you had time, there'd be little point in holding off the prep and coming back later; the patient would probably get an erection again, with even more embarrassment than before.

* Erections during catheter change

A burn patient in his early 20s develops an erection each time I change his external catheter. Should I reprimand him for this, or just ignore it?

Neither. The erection is almost certainly an involuntary response to the handling of his penis for the catheter change. Since he's likely to be embarrassed by it, you can make the situation more relaxed by discussing how it comes about.

Let him know that you realize it's a reflex reaction, like a blink. His penis stiffens and rises because blood engorges the corpora cavernosa, the balloon-like pair of chambers comprising the bulk of the erect penis, and the corpus spongiosum, the spongy tissue forming the ridge along the bottom.

You might point out that men don't have to be sexually aroused to develop an erection. Merely touching his penis or another genital zone can trigger a man's pudendal nerves. These run to his lower spinal cord, where a nerve center relaxes muscles in the walls of arteries supplying his penis. When the arteries expand, increased blood flows into the spongy tissue. This in turn compresses penile veins, sustaining the erection.

From very slight tactile stimulation, a patient can develop an erection in less than 10 seconds. With the cessation of stimuli, the arterial muscles soon contract. Blood flow to the penis is restricted, venous compression eases, the engorged areas empty, and the penis once more becomes flaccid.

* Is an MD's permission needed for sex talks?

Does a med-surg nurse need a physician's permission to discuss his patient's sexual worries?

Not unless you're specifically instructed to avoid the subject. As a nurse, you can address the sexual needs of patients just as you can their dietary needs. The information and advice you give may keep a simple concern from escalating into a major problem. Further, you're in a good position to serve as a role model, reflecting to the patient and family your comfort with sexual matters.

Your professional judgment will ordinarily tell you if a sexual discussion is going beyond your ability to handle it. Then, as with any other problem in nursing, you need merely say, "I'm not sure I have the answer. Let me find out for you."

* Promoting sex education for colleagues

I learn a lot at clinical conferences on sexuality. But when I come back to my hospital, I find that my colleagues are cool to the whole subject. Despite my arguments, I can't convince them of the importance of the sexual aspects of patient care. How do you suggest that I persuade them otherwise?

For starters, we suggest that you refrain from arguing. There's no way you can talk another person into changing longstanding sexual attitudes. Indeed, angry exchanges are more likely to make your colleagues defensive than to gain their cooperation.

Instead, try to assume the position of a role model. Work at becoming ever more comfortable with your own sexuality and that of your patients. And put your knowledge into practice quietly and competently.

We'd also suggest that you examine your motives for being so vehement with your colleagues. We've seen some nurses become almost evangelical with their new insights into sexuality. And we've seen others who suddenly feel liberated—and can't resist raising the eyebrows of their traditional-minded colleagues. Don't *overdo* your enthusiasm.

You'll find it's more constructive to proceed slowly and diplomatically. You might remind yourself that it was not very long ago (in 1966) that *Human Sexual Response*, Masters' and Johnson's landmark report of their physiological studies, was published. Small wonder that some of your most conscientious, skillful colleagues may still be dubious about the subject.

*

Selected Bibliography

*

THESE LISTS of titles have been prepared in cooperation with the professional staff of the Sex Information and Education Council of the United States (SIECUS).*

Much of the material here is of special interest to health professionals. In addition are listed many items you might care to recommend to patients, their families, and other members of the general public, including teachers, clergy, youth leaders, and librarians. Titles were chosen that span a variety of viewpoints at different levels of sophistication.

With few exceptions, these materials are included in the noncirculating collection at the SIECUS Resource Center and Library, New York University, 51 West Fourth St., New York, N.Y. 10003.

For the latest updated editions of SIECUS bibliographies, send $1 and a stamped, self-addressed business size envelope to SIECUS, 80 Fifth Ave., Suite 801, New York, N.Y. 10011.

From the same address you can also get information about SIECUS publications and membership. SIECUS is an excellent source of current information in the field of human sexuality. Other major organizations in the field include:

• American Association of Sex Educators, Counselors, and Therapists, 11 Dupont Circle, N.W., Washington, D.C. 20036.

• Planned Parenthood Federation of America, 810 Seventh Ave., New York, N.Y. 10019.

• Society for the Scientific Study of Sex, P.O. Box 29795, Philadelphia, Pa.,19117.

FOR PROFESSIONALS

*

Textbooks

FOR USE WITH ADOLESCENTS

Learning About Sex: The Contemporary Guide for Young Adults
Gary F. Kelly
Without neglecting basic factual information, focuses on attitudes and the process of sexual decision making. Teacher's manual available. *Barron's Educational Series (1977), 113 Crossways Park Dr., Woodbury, N.Y. 11797.*

Masculinity and Feminity *Revised Edition*
Elizabeth Winship, Frank Caparulo, and Vivian Harlin
Basic high school text covering factual information as well as attitudes and emotions. *Houghton Mifflin (1978), 1 Beacon St., Boston, Mass. 02107.*

Modern Human Sexuality
Burt Saxon and Peter Kelman
Effective text for human sexuality courses aimed at early adolescents, stressing sexual responsibility. *Houghton Mifflin (1976), 1 Beacon St., Boston, Mass. 02107.*

COLLEGE TEXTS

Becoming a Sexual Person
Robert T. Francoeur
John Wiley & Sons (1982), 605 Third Ave., New York, N.Y. 10158.

Human Sexuality
William H. Masters, Virginia E. Johnson, and Robert C. Kolodny
Little, Brown & Co. (1982), 34 Beacon St., Boston, Mass. 02106.

Human Sexuality *Fourth Edition*
James L. McCary and Stephen P. McCary
Wadsworth (1982), 7625 Empire Dr., Florence, Ky. 41042.

Human Sexuality: Making Responsible Decisions
Linda Brower Meeks and Philip Heit
Holt, Rinehart & Winston (1982), 383 Madison Ave., New York, N.Y. 10017.

Our Sexuality *Second Edition*
Robert Crooks and Karla Baur
Benjamin/Cummings (1983), Sand Hill Rd., Menlo Park, Calif. 94025.

TEXTS FOR HEALTH PROFESSIONALS

(See also Sexuality and the Disabled, page 153.)

Human Sexuality: A Health Practitioner's Text *Second Edition*
Richard Green, ed.
A well-integrated collection of essays, written by experts, designed to increase health practitioners' competence and skill in the management of sexual concerns and problems. *Williams & Wilkins (1979), 428 East Preston St., Baltimore, Md. 21202.*

Human Sexuality: A Nursing Perspective
Rosemarie Hogan
Appleton-Century-Crofts (1980), 25 Van Zant St., East Norwalk, Conn. 06855.

Human Sexuality in Health and Illness *Second Edition*
Nancy Fugate Woods
C. V. Mosby (1979), 11830 Westline Industrial Dr., St. Louis, Mo. 63141.

Human Sexuality in Nursing Process
Elizabeth M. Lion
John Wiley & Sons (1982), 605 Third Ave., New York, N.Y. 10158.

Sexuality: A Nursing Perspective
Fern H. Mins and Melinda Swenson
McGraw-Hill (1979), 1221 Avenue of the Americas, New York, N.Y. 10020.

Textbook of Human Sexuality for Nurses
Robert C. Kolodny, William H. Masters, Virginia E. Johnson, and Mae E. Biggs
Comprehensive work on human sexuality as a clinical science for the nursing profession, from basic sexual anatomy to discussions of medical and surgical conditions in each of the major body systems and their biologic and/or psychosocial impacts on sexuality. Includes effects of drugs and of endocrine disorders on sexual functioning. *Little, Brown (1979), 34 Beacon St., Boston, Mass. 02106.*

Textbook of Sexual Medicine
Robert C. Kolodny, William H. Masters, and Virginia E. Johnson
Designed to meet the needs of primary-care providers, medical or surgical specialists, and sex therapists working with patients and clients who have sexual problems. *Little, Brown (1979), 34 Beacon St., Boston, Mass. 02106.*

Basic Resources

Handbook of Sexology
John Money and Herman Musaph, eds.
Designed to encourage sexology as a medical subspecialty. Comprehensive volume of what is currently known in the field of sexuality. Contains 108 chapters by

102 authors—almost half of whom are from outside the U.S. *Excerpta Medica/Elsevier North-Holland (1977), 52 Vanderbilt Ave., New York, N.Y. 10017.*

Human Sexual Response
William H. Masters and Virginia E. Johnson
Report of the laboratory research and clinical findings concerning sexual response of men and women during various types of sexual activity, during pregnancy, and in the later years. Contains the most definitive physiological data concerning sexual response so far developed. *Little, Brown (1966), 34 Beacon St., Boston, Mass. 02106.*

Human Sexuality: Methods and Materials for the Education, Family Life, and Health Professions *Volume I: An Annotated Guide to the Audiovisuals*
Ronald S. Daniel
Annotated listings of 3100 audiovisuals categorized into 28 basic topic areas. Unique and valuable resource for educators, counselors, and therapists. Supplements planned. *Heuristicus (1979), 401 Tolbert St., Brea, Calif. 92621.*

The Kinsey Data: Marginal Tabulations of the 1938–1963 Interviews Conducted by the Institute for Sex Research
Paul H. Gebhard and Alan B. Johnson
Important revision of and supplement to the previously published Kinsey data. Includes 45 pages of text with 580 statistical tables. Offers a valuable opportunity for researchers to compare their current findings with Kinsey's figures for an earlier generation. *W. B. Saunders (1979), West Washington Sq., Philadelphia, Pa. 19105.*

The Selective Guide to Audiovisuals for Mental Health and Family Life Education *Fourth Edition*
Mental Health Materials Center
Excellent resource for selection and evaluation of audiovisuals in the fields of mental health and family life education. More than 400 listings, arranged by subject. Revised edition in progress. *Marquis Academic Media (1979), 200 East Ohio St., Chicago, Ill. 60611.*

The Selective Guide to Publications for Mental Health and Family Life Education *Fourth Edition*
Mental Health Materials Center
Invaluable resource for selection and evaluation of materials in the fields of mental health and family life education. More than 470 entries, arranged by subject. Revised edition in progress. *Marquis Academic Media (1979), 200 East Ohio St., Chicago, Ill. 60611.*

Sex and Health: A Practical Guide to Sexual Medicine
Armando DeMoya, Dorothy DeMoya, Martha E. Lewis, and Howard R. Lewis
Organized into about 200 alphabetical entries, this book presents practical information derived from sexual medicine, dealing with how sexual activities can affect physical health; how medical conditions may influence sexual functioning; how

medications and other drugs may impair sexual functioning and fertility; how people with disabilities and illnesses can find sexual fulfillment; how to decide among birth control methods; and how to avoid, recognize, and treat sexually transmitted diseases. *Stein & Day (1983), Scarborough House, Briarcliff Manor, N.Y. 10510.*

The Sex Atlas *New Popular Reference Edition*
Erwin J. Haeberle
A comprehensive source book of basic textual and pictorial information on human sexuality for college students, parents, and professionals. May also be used as a text. *Continuum (1981), 575 Lexington Ave., New York, N.Y. 10022.*

Sex in History
Reay Tannahill
Well-written, frank exploration of human sexuality through the ages, containing a wealth of relevant information. *Stein & Day (1980), Scarborough House, Briarcliff Manor, N.Y. 10510.*

Sex: The Facts, the Acts, and Your Feelings
Michael Carrera
Comprehensive, accurate, and easy-to-understand information about sexuality presented in a nonjudgmental tone, imparting values concerned with people and relationships. Also useful as a text. *Crown (1981), 1 Park Ave., New York, N.Y. 10016.*

Teenage Pregnancy: The Problem That Hasn't Gone Away
The Alan Guttmacher Institute
Well-documented report, presenting a comprehensive summary of the current teenage pregnancy epidemic. Essential resource for all those providing services to sexually active teenagers, and for everyone concerned about the problem. *The Alan Guttmacher Institute (1981), 360 Park Ave. South, New York, N.Y. 10010.*

*

Sex Research

The Frontiers of Sex Research
Vern Bullough, ed.
Provocative volume reviewing with fresh insights the frontiers of the sexual revolution. *Prometheus (1979), 700 East Amherst St., Buffalo, N.Y. 14215.*

Sex Research: Bibliographies from the Institute for Sex Research
Joan S. Brewer and Rod W. Wright, comps.
Valuable research and reference tool; 4000 citations arranged by 11 major subject headings. *Oryx (1979), 2214 North Central at Encanto, Phoenix, Ariz. 85004.*

The Sex Researchers *Revised Edition*
Edward M. Brecher
Selective review of research, with an enthusiastic, human, and liberal approach to sexual behavior. Revised edition contains 1978 epilogue. *Specific (1979), 1523 Franklin St., San Francisco, Calif. 94109.*

Taking a Sex History: Interviewing and Recording
Wardell B. Pomeroy, Carol C. Flax, and Connie Christine Wheeler
The first published guide to the famous and pioneering Kinsey sex interview technique, explaining in depth virtually all the questioning and coding skills a professional requires to compile a detailed, accurate, confidential sex history that defines an individual's sexual attitudes and behaviors. *The Free Press, Macmillan (1982), 855 Third Ave., New York, N.Y. 10022.*

*

Sexuality and The Life Cycle

CHILDHOOD

Childhood and Sexuality: Proceedings of the International Symposium
Jean-Marc Samson, ed.
Papers presented at a unique and important conference held at the University of Quebec in 1979. Includes state-of-the-art reports by the most noted experts on this subject. *Editions Etudes Vivantes (1980), 6700 chemin Côte de Liesse, Saint-Laurent, Montreal, Quebec H4T 1E3, Canada.*

Children and Sex: New Findings, New Perspectives
Larry L. Constantine and Floyd M. Martinston, eds.
Deals seriously with sex and sexuality as essential phenomena of childhood. Human sexuality is seen as a unitary phenomenon with the sexuality of childhood, youth, maturity, and aging being parts of a continuum. Coverage takes into account the full spectrum of disciplines from anthropology and sociology through psychology, social work, psychiatry, and psychoanalysis. *Little, Brown (1981), 34 Beacon St., Boston, Mass. 02106.*

Children's Sexual Thinking
Ronald Goldman and Juliette Goldman
Based on interviews with hundreds of children aged five to 15 in North America, England, Sweden, and Australia. Topics examined include how children perceive aging, parental roles, gender identity, sex roles, conception and birth, contraception, marriage, and nudity. Findings are discussed in light of various developmental theories, and the implications for sex education are examined. *Routledge and Kegan Paul (1982), 9 Park St., Boston, Mass 02108.*

Family Life and Sexual Learning: A Study of the Role of Parents in the Sexual Learning of Children *Volume 1: Summary Report*
Project on Human Sexual Development
A major study of more than 1400 parents of three- to 11-year-old children in Cleveland, Ohio. Documents difficulty parents have in communicating with their children about sex. Three companion volumes available. *Project on Human Sexual Development (1978), 601 Larsen Hall, 13 Appian Way, Cambridge, Mass. 02138.*

ADOLESCENCE AND YOUNG ADULTHOOD

Adolescent Pregnancy: Perspectives for the Health Professional
Peggy B. Smith and David M. Mumford, eds.
A collection of articles by professionals in a variety of health fields, presenting the social, emotional, legal, medical, and educational aspects of adolescent pregnancy. *G. K. Hall (1980), 70 Lincoln St., Boston, Mass. 02111.*

Adolescent Sexuality in a Changing American Society: Social and Psychological Perspectives
Catherine S. Chilman
Responsible and comprehensive review of pertinent literature up to 1976. *Superintendent of Documents U.S. Government Printing Office (1978), Washington, D.C. 20402.*

Growing Up Sexual
Eleanor Morrison, Kay Starks, Cynda Hyndman, and Nina Ronzio
Unique view of patterns of human sexual development based on anonymous autobiographical papers by students in a college human sexuality course. *Brooks/Cole (1980), 555 Abrego, Monterey, Calif. 93940.*

Premarital Sexuality: Attitudes, Relationships, Behavior
John DeLameter and Patricia MacCorquodale
Examines the influence of psychological, social, and interpersonal variables on the development of human sexual expression and points to a variety of implications and conclusions about the nature of premarital sexual behavior. *University of Wisconsin Press (1979), 114 North Murray St., Madison, Wis. 53715.*

The Sexual Adolescent: Communicating with Teenagers About Sex
Second Edition
Sol Gordon, Peter Scales, and Kathleen Everly
Thoughtful discussion about adolescent sexual behavior, stressing the importance of sexual responsibility and communication. Useful appendix of additional resources. *Ed-U (1979), P.O. Box 583, Fayetteville, N.Y. 13066.*

Sexual Unfolding: Sexual Development and Sex Therapies in Late Adolescence
Lorna Sarrel and Philip Sarrel
An important book for those interested in their capacity to deal positively with the sexuality and sexual mores and adjustment of young adults. *Little, Brown (1979), 34 Beacon St., Boston, Mass. 02106.*

Teenage Pregnancy in a Family Context: Implications for Policy
Theodora Ooms, ed.
Important book of readings in light of attempts by the U.S. government to deal with adolescent sexual activity, contraception, pregnancy, abortion, and parenthood via greater parental involvement. *Temple University Press (1981), Broad and Oxford, Philadelphia, Pa. 19122.*

Teenage Sexuality, Pregnancy, and Childbearing
Frank F. Furstenberg Jr., Richard Lincoln, and Jane Menken, eds.
Excellent compilation of 28 articles reprinted from *Family Planning Perspectives*, with introductions summarizing major themes and research findings. Useful for professionals engaged in research, program development, or direct services. *University of Pennsylvania Press (1981), 3933 Walnut St., Philadelphia, Pa. 19104.*

MATURE ADULTHOOD

Changing Perspectives on Menopause
Ann M. Voda, Myra Dinnerstein, and Sheryl R. O'Donnell, eds.
A collection of 27 papers presented at the Third Interdisciplinary Research Conference on Menopause held in 1979. All but three of the contributors are women. An outstanding interdisciplinary approach, written from the viewpoint that menopause is a normal stage of life. *University of Texas Press (1981), Box 7819, University Station, Austin, Texas 78712.*

Love and Sex After Sixty: A Guide for Men and Women for Their Later Years
Robert N. Butler and Myrna I. Lewis
A practical book giving older people guidance in enjoying—to whatever degree and in whatever way they wish—the satisfactions of physical sex and pleasurable sensuality. *Harper & Row (1977), 10 East 53rd St., New York, N.Y. 10022.*

The Starr-Weiner Report on Sex and Sexuality in the Mature Years
Bernard D. Starr and Marcella Bakur Weiner
Based on responses from more than 800 individuals older than 60, the majority of whom are sexually active. Includes information on attitudes toward oral sex, masturbation, living together outside of marriage, and nudity. *Stein & Day (1981), Scarborough House, Briarcliff Manor, N.Y. 10510.*

Female and Male Sexuality

The Hite Report
Shere Hite
Based on responses to in-depth questionnaires returned by some 3000 women. A provocative and revealing study that examines the subject of female sexuality from the inside. Makes extensive use of direct quotes to illustrate the various topics. *Macmillan (1976), 866 Third Ave., New York, N.Y. 10022. Dell, 1 Dag Hammarskjold Plaza, New York, N.Y. 10017.*

The Hite Report on Male Sexuality
Shere Hite
Based on questionnaire responses from more than 7000 men. Depicts the enormous variety and diversity of male sexual expressions and attitudes and presents provocative ideas about the nature of sexual intercourse and other forms of sexual behavior. *Alfred A. Knopf (1981), 201 East 50th St., New York, N.Y. 10022.*

Sexual Behavior in the Human Female
Alfred C. Kinsey, Wardell B. Pomeroy, Clyde E. Martin, and Paul Gebhard
The companion study to the male volume but done with more statistical sophistication. Contrasts data on male and female sexual response in addition to the findings on female sexual behavior. *W. B. Saunders (1953), West Washington Sq., Philadelphia, Pa. 19105.*

Sexual Behavior in the Human Male
Alfred C. Kinsey, Wardell B. Pomeroy, and Clyde E. Martin
The first of the famous Kinsey Reports and a pioneering study of male sexual behavior. Demonstrated statistically for the first time how wide the gap had become between officially sanctioned and actual sexual behavior in our society. *W. B. Saunders (1948), West Washington Sq., Philadelphia. Pa. 19105.*

Women: Sex and Sexuality
Catherine R. Stimpson and Ethel Spector Person, eds.
A collection of articles from the feminist journal *Signs*, discussing aspects of female sexuality from a variety of viewpoints. Juxtaposes ideas from the behavioral sciences with those from the humanities. *University of Chicago Press (1980), 5801 Ellis Ave., Chicago, Ill. 60637.*

Women's Sexual Development: Outer Form and Inner Space
Martha Kirkpatrick, ed.
These papers, written from a variety of theoretical perspectives, illustrate the complexity of the subject of female sexual development and suggest areas for further investigation. *Plenum (1980), 233 Spring St., New York, N.Y. 10013.*

Gender Identity and Sex Roles

Man & Woman, Boy & Girl
John Money and Anke A. Ehrhardt
An authoritative and technical treatment of the differentiation and dimorphism of gender identity from conception to maturity. Clarifies the interaction between genetics and environment, discusses the research on the development of gender identity, and provides insights into homosexuality, transsexualism, sexual anomalies, and transvestism. *The Johns Hopkins University Press (1973), Baltimore, Md. 21218.*

The Psychobiology of Sex Differences and Sex Roles
Jacquelynne E. Parsons, ed.
Critical assessment of biological research and theory on sexual dimorphism and women's life cycles. Useful for bringing to the attention of social scientists current knowledge concerning these biological issues. *McGraw-Hill (1980), 1221 Avenue of the Americas, New York, N.Y. 10020.*

The Psychology of Sex Differences
Eleanor Maccoby and Carol Jacklin
Reviews and evaluates the experimental and theoretical literature on psychological sex differences. After surveying studies dealing with intellectual, perceptual, learning and memory, achievement, sexual, emotional, and activity differences between females and males, the authors discuss the theories offered to explain these differences. *Stanford University Press (1974), Stanford, Calif. 94305.*

Sex Errors of the Body
John Money
Discusses various types of anomalies in development, explaining their causes, their psychosexual effects, and the necessary sex education to help the individual achieve successful sexual attitudes and functioning or to provide supportive counseling. *The Johns Hopkins University Press (1968), Baltimore, Md. 21218.*

Sexual Signatures: On Being a Man or a Woman
John Money and Patricia Tucker
An interpretation of the more technical *Man & Woman, Boy & Girl.* Summarizes research on the process of gender identity differentiation in individuals and the possible genetic, hormonal, or psychosocial influences that result in the taking of different pathways toward sexual identity. Provides a detailed account of just how we respond to the plethora of forces impinging on us from conception onward. *Little, Brown (1975), 34 Beacon St., Boston, Mass. 02106.*

Transsexuality in the Male: The Spectrum of Gender Dysphoria
Erwin K. Koranyi
Useful addition to literature of transsexual theory and practice in medicine. Supports the therapeutic approach in favor of sex reassignment. *Charles C Thomas (1980), 2600 South First St., Springfield, Ill. 62717.*

Transvestites and Transsexuals: Mixed Views
Deborah H. Feinbloom
The sociologist author interviewed, observed, and corresponded with scores of transvestites and transsexuals to gather her data and draw her conclusions. A welcome appendix addresses the problem of ethics in carrying out such research. *Dell (1977), 1 Dag Hammarskjold Plaza, New York, N.Y. 10017.*

*

Sexual Behaviors

The Bisexual Option
Fred Klein
Useful addition to the limited amount of literature available concerning research on this topic. *Arbor House (1979), 235 East 45th St., New York, N.Y. 10017. Berkley Publishing, 200 Madison Ave., New York, N.Y. 10016.*

Homosexual Behavior: A Modern Reappraisal
Judd Marmor, ed.
A well-balanced, extremely informative, and excellently written consideration of homosexuality. Highly recommended. *Basic (1980), 10 East 53rd St., New York, N.Y. 10022.*

Sexual Preference: Its Development in Men and Women
Alan P. Bell, Martin S. Weinberg, and Sue Kiefer Hammersmith
Based on data from interviews with approximately 1500 individuals, this study charts the development of both homosexuality and heterosexuality among males and females and statistically tests popular notions about the causes of homosexuality. Main volume presents the questions and quotes typical answers. The complete sets of diagrams and tables are given in the *Statistical Appendix. Indiana University Press (1981), 10th & Morton, Bloomington, Ind. 47401.*

*

Sex Education

An Analysis of U.S. Sex Education Programs and Evaluation Methods
Mathtech
Five-volume study. Most useful for sex educators is Volume 1, which reviews the literature on the effects of sex education programs, identifies important features and outcomes of programs, selects and summarizes excellent school and non-school programs, and analyzes state guidelines for sex education. *National Technical Information Service (1979), U.S. Department of Commerce, Springfield, Va. 22161.*

Childhood Sexual Learning: The Unwritten Curriculum
Elizabeth J. Roberts, ed.
Explores the many areas in which learning about sexuality takes place, including the family, school, television, social services, peers, and religion. Examines the assumptions about sexuality underlying institutional policies and practices. *Ballinger (1980), 17 Dunster St., Harvard Sq., Cambridge, Mass. 02138.*

Dealing with Questions About Sex
Arlene Uslander and Caroline Weiss
Written for sex education teachers. A down-to-earth and lively handbook. *Pitman Learning (1975), 6 Davis Dr., Belmont, Calif. 94002.*

Journal of School Health, April 1981 Special Issue: Sex Education in the Public Schools
Guy Parcel and Sol Gordon, issue eds.
Excellent collection of articles supporting sex education in the school setting. Especially valuable as a resource for communities and school personnel in developing sex education programs. *American School Health Association, P.O. Box 708, Kent, Ohio 44240.*

The Professional Training and Preparation of Sex Educators
American Association of Sex Educators, Counselors, and Therapists
A booklet prepared by AASECT's Training and Standards Committee that outlines the scope of knowledge, personal qualities, and professional skills essential for anyone working in this field. *American Association of Sex Educators, Counselors, and Therapists (1972), 11 Dupont Circle, N.W., Washington, D.C. 20036.*

Schools and Parents—Partners in Sex Education *Public Affairs Pamphlet #581*
Sol Gordon and Irving R. Dickman
Booklet stressing the importance of including parents as partners in sex education. Includes a model curriculum. *Public Affairs Committee (1980), 381 Park Ave. South, New York, N.Y. 10016.*

Sex Education Books for Young Adults 1892–1979
Patricia J. Campbell
A spectrum of sex education books published for young adults during an 87-year period, ending with an annotated bibliography of more recent selections. Useful for historical perspective. *R. R. Bowker (1979), 1180 Avenue of the Americas, New York, N.Y. 10036.*

Sex Education for Adolescents: A Bibliography of Low-Cost Materials
Criteria used for selection: appropriateness to adolescents in readability; cost of $6.00 or less; and values perspective responsibly represented in contemporary terms but without limitation as to position on the conservative-liberal spectrum. *American Library Association Order Department (1980), 50 East Huron St., Chicago, Ill. 60611.*

Sex Education for the Health Professional: A Curriculum Guide
Norman Rosenzweig and F. Paul Pearsall, eds.
A highly informative collection representing diversified points of view about both the subject matter and the teaching styles required for a wide variety of audiences. *Grune & Stratton (1978), 111 Fifth Ave., New York, N.Y. 10003.*

Sex Education in the Eighties: The Challenge of Healthy Sexual Evolution
Lorna Brown, ed.
Opening with a historical perspective on sex education in the U.S., the contributors go on to present an overview of the field. There are chapters covering the issue from the standpoint of the family, society at large, and education for professionals. Closes with predictions for future developments. *Plenum (1981), 233 Spring St., New York, N.Y. 10013.*

The Sexual and Gender Development of Young Children: The Role of the Educator
Evelyn K. Oremland and Jerome D. Oremland, eds.
Enriching for educators generally, and an absolute must for sex educators. Multidisciplinary perspectives by outstanding authorities on sexual and gender development in children. *Ballinger (1977), 17 Dunster St., Harvard Sq., Cambridge, Mass. 02138.*

Winning the Battle for Sex Education
Irving R. Dickman
Designed to help parents, teachers, administrators, and other members of a community effectively organize support for a public school sex education program. Includes answers to the 20 questions most often asked about such programs. *SIECUS (1982), 80 Fifth Ave., Suite 801, New York, N.Y. 10011.*

Autobiography, Fiction For Sex Education

Are You There, God? It's Me, Margaret
Judy Blume
Reassuring story about preadolescent girls as they face the physical changes that usually accompany puberty, as well as peer pressure. *Bradbury (1970), 2 Overhill Rd., Scarsdale, N.Y. 10583. Dell, 1 Dag Hammarskjold Plaza, New York, N.Y. 10017.*

The Best Little Boy in the World
John Reid
A story of coming to terms with being gay, told with warmth and humor. *Ballantine (1976), 400 Hahn Rd., Westminster, Md. 21157.*

Forever
Judy Blume
Its reception by adolescents has made this book a classic. A story of first love with explicit passages about the adolescents' sexual experiences. *Bradbury (1975), 2 Overhill Rd., Scarsdale, N.Y. 10583. Pocket Books, Simon & Schuster, 1230 Avenue of the Americas, New York, N.Y. 10020.*

Patience and Sarah
Isabel Miller
A story set in early 19th century America, about the resourcefulness and love of a lesbian couple who establish their own farm. *Fawcett Crest (1979), 1515 Broadway, New York, N.Y. 10036.*

Reflections of a Rock Lobster: A Story About Growing Up Gay
Aaron Fricke
Moving autobiographical account of a young man coming to terms with his homosexuality and coming out to his family and high school peers. *Alyson (1981), P.O. Box 2783, Dept. B2, Boston, Mass. 02208.*

Rubyfruit Jungle
Rita Mae Brown
A down-to-earth, vibrant story of a lesbian's journey from early childhood to adulthood. *Bantam (1977), 666 Fifth Ave., New York, N.Y. 10019.*

*

Sex Counseling and Therapy

The Behavioral Treatment of Sexual Problems *Volume 1: Brief Therapy (Revised Edition) Volume II: Intensive Therapy*
Jack S. Annon
Volume I outlines Dr. Annon's theoretical model for approaching sexual problems, referred to as PLISSIT (permission, limited information, selected suggestion, and intensive therapy). Volume II is both a practical book with detailed explanation as to how various interpretations were made and a theoretical book with explanation as to why the author took the routes he did in treating sexual problems. *Harper & Row (1976), 10 East 53rd St., New York, N.Y. 10022.*

Counseling Lesbian Women and Gay Men: A Life-Issues Approach
A Elfin Moses and Robert O. Hawkins Jr.
Brings together clarity in theory, sensitivity in understanding the experiences of being gay, and practical suggestions in working with gay concerns. Helpful not only to those counseling gay people, but also to anyone who is interested in a deeper understanding of human nature and interpersonal dynamics. *C. V. Mosby (1981), 11830 Westline Industrial Dr., St., Louis, Mo. 63141.*

Disorders of Sexual Desire and Other New Concepts and Techniques in Sex Therapy
Helen Singer Kaplan
Detailed case studies illuminating the dysfunction involving inhibition of sexual desire. Presents psychosexual therapy developed by the author. *Brunner/Mazel (1979), 19 Union Sq. West, New York, N.Y. 10003.*

Handbook of Sex Therapy
Joseph LoPiccolo and Leslie LoPiccolo, eds.
Practical handbook providing up-to-date information about a wide variety of new techniques and specific methodologies. *Plenum (1978), 233 Spring St., New York, N.Y. 10013.*

Human Sexual Inadequacy
William H. Masters and Virginia E. Johnson
Based on authors' landmark research, presents findings for the treatment of impotence, ejaculatory disorders, inadequate female response, vaginismus, dyspareunia, and sexual problems of aging. A basic resource for therapists and counselors. *Little, Brown (1970), 34 Beacon St., Boston, Mass. 02106, Bantam (1980), 666 Fifth Ave., New York, N.Y. 10019.*

Impotence: Physiological, Psychological, and Surgical Diagnosis and Treatment
Gorm Wagner and Richard Green
After a brief series of case histories designed to illustrate some of the points, the reader is lead through a series of chapters on physiology, diagnosis, and disease processes that can cause sexual dysfunction. Both a gem of brevity and a definitive work on the topic. *Plenum (1981), 233 Spring St., New York, N.Y. 10013.*

Lifelong Sexual Vigor: How to Avoid and Overcome Impotence
Marvin B. Brooks and Sally West Brooks
An important work and comprehensive review on the subject of erectile dysfunction, presented in fluid prose style. *Doubleday (1981). 501 Franklin Ave., Garden City, N.Y. 11530.*

The New Sex Therapy
Helen Singer Kaplan
A comprehensive and eclectic approach to the treatment of sexual dysfunction, integrating psychoanalytic and a number of other techniques. Includes an appendix of 39 illustrative case studies and tables of the effects of various drugs on male and female sexual function. *Brunner/Mazel (1974), 19 Union Sq. West, New York, N.Y. 10003.*

The Prevention of Sexual Disorders: Issues and Approaches
C. Brandon Qualls, John P. Wincze, and David H. Barlow, eds.
Well-integrated contributions concerning the important need for preventive programs in maintaining sexual health. Confronts readers with the importance of

going beyond "issues and approaches" and working toward action. *Plenum (1978), 233 Spring St., New York, N.Y. 10013.*

Principles and Practice of Sex Therapy
Sandra R. Leiblum and Lawrence A. Pervin, eds.
Comprehensive updating of treatment methods and efficacy studies in sex therapy. *Guilford (1980), 200 Park Ave. South, New York, N.Y. 10003.*

The Professional Training and Preparation of Sex Counselors and Sex Therapists
American Association of Sex Educators, Counselors, and Therapists
Emphasizes counseling principles and procedures and outlines the scope of sex counseling and the requisite training. *American Association of Sex Educators, Counselors, and Therapists (1973), 11 Dupont Circle, N.W., Washington, D.C. 20036.*

Sexual Medicine and Counseling in Office Practice: A Comprehensive Treatment Guide
Dennis J. Munjack and L. Jerome Oziel
First half covers the fundamental principles of sex counseling, including sexual history taking, physiology of human sexual response, and the problems of sexuality in the course of various systemic disorders and aging. The second half outlines advanced sexual counseling for male and female dysfunction.Useful for all types of physicians and therapists. *Little, Brown (1980), 34 Beacon St., Boston, Mass. 02106.*

Sexual Problems in Medical Practice
Harold I. Lief, ed.
Represents a major step toward filling the educational vacuum that exists in the majority of medical schools and residency training programs whose graduate physicians are inadequately prepared to deal with sexual problems. *American Medical Association (1981), 535 North Dearborn St., Chicago, Ill. 60610.*

Women Discover Orgasm: A Therapist's Guide to a New Treatment Approach
Lonnie Barbach
A new approach through a group treatment method for dealing with orgasmic dysfunction in women. *Macmillan (1980), 866 Third Ave., New York, N.Y. 10022.*

*

Sexuality and the Disabled

Body Image, Self-Esteem, and Sexuality in Cancer Patients
J. M. Vaeth, R. C. Blomberg, and L. Adler, eds.
The conference on which this outstanding book is based was a first in the specific area of cancer and its possible effects on sexuality and self-esteem in patients of all ages. *S. Karger (1980), 150 Fifth Ave., New York, N.Y. 10011.*

Family Planning Services for Disabled People: A Manual for Service Providers
Ebon Research Systems
Excellent resource that provides guidance for training staff to work with disabled persons, making clinics barrier-free, and offering services related to specific disabilities. Includes a chart of disabling conditions and their effects on reproduction and contraception. *National Clearinghouse for Family Planning Information (1980), P.O. Box 2225, Rockville, Md. 20852.*

Female Sexuality Following Spinal Cord Injury
Elle Friedman Becker
Offers an opportunity to understand the struggle of a quadriplegic or paraplegic woman in a world that represses and defines her sexual expression and identity, and to learn what disabled people look to from the professional community and from their families and friends. *Cheever (1978), P.O. Box 700, Bloomington, Ill. 61701.*

Guidelines for Training in Sexuality and the Mentally Handicapped
Winifred Kempton and Rose Forman
Not a textbook, but a proposed training program for those working with staff, aides, or parents involved with the mentally handicapped. *Planned Parenthood of Southeastern Pennsylvania (1976), 1220 Samson St., Philadelphia, Pa. 19107.*

Human Sexuality and Rehabilitation Medicine: Sexual Functioning Following Spinal Cord Injury
Ami Ska'ked, ed.
Fifteen chapters for health-care professionals who deal with spinal cord injury as well as other disabilities, to help people adjust to their problems. *Williams & Wilkins (1981), 428 East Preston St., Baltimore, Md. 21202.*

Human Sexuality in Health and Illness *Second Edition*
Nancy Fugate Woods
Examines the biophysical nature of human sexuality, sexual health and health care (including preventive and restorative intervention and sexual dysfunction), and clinical aspects of human sexuality in such concerns as chronic illness, paraplegia, and adaptation to changed body image. *C. V. Mosby (1979), 11830 Westline Industrial Dr., St. Louis, Mo. 63141.*

Human Sexuality in Physical and Mental Illnesses and Disabilities: An Annotated Bibliography
Ami Ska'ked
Excellent resource for all those who provide help with sexual and sex-related problems of the ill, aged, and disabled. *Indiana University Press (1979), Tenth & Morton, Bloomington, Ind. 47405.*

The Sensuous Wheeler: Sexual Adjustment for the Spinal Cord Injured
Barry J. Rabin
Informal, positive treatment of the subject, stressing the sharing of sexual responsibilities and vulnerabilities. *Multi Media Resource Center (1980), 1525 Franklin St., San Francisco, Calif. 94109.*

Sex Education and Counseling of Special Groups: The Mentally and Physically Handicapped, Ill, and Elderly *Second Edition*
Warren R. Johnson and Winifred Kempton
Deals with problem areas in sex education and counseling of handicapped persons and points out danger of losing the individual behind group labels. Offers suggestions for dealing with sex-related topics from masturbation to abortion. *Charles C Thomas (1981), 2600 South First St., Springfield, Ill. 62717.*

Sex Education for Persons with Disabilities That Hinder Learning: A Teacher's Guide
Winifred Kempton
Invaluable resource for instructors on human sexuality for students with learning problems, stressing the need to integrate sexuality with every facet of human experience. *Planned Parenthood of Southeastern Pennsylvania (1975), 1220 Sansom St., Philadelphia. Pa. 19107.*

Sex, Society, and the Disabled: A Developmental Inquiry into Roles, Reactions, and Responsibilities
Isabel P. Robinault
An excellent resource, presenting a chronological discussion of the sexuality of people with physical disabilities. *Harper & Row (1978), 10 East 53rd St., New York, N.Y. 10022.*

Sexual Consequences of Disability
Alex Comfort
Useful reference for professionals in sexual counseling of disabled people. *Stickley (1978), West Washington Sq., Philadelphia, Pa. 19106.*

Sexual Rehabilitation of the Urologic Cancer Patient
Andrew C. von Eschenbach and Dorothy Rodriquez, eds.
This collection of articles is derived from papers presented at a 1979 seminar at the University of Texas in Houston. A valuable book for any individual involved in the total care of patients with urologic cancer. *G. K. Hall (1981), 70 Lincoln St., Boston, Mass. 02111.*

Sexuality and Cancer
Jean M. Stoklosa, David G. Bullard, Ernest H. Rosenbaum, and Isadora R. Rosenbaum
Sensitively written discussion with useful sections on ostomy, laryngectomy, and mastectomy. *Bull (1979), Box 208, Palo Alto, Calif. 94302.*

Sexuality and Disability: A Bibliography of Resources Available to Purchase
Leigh Hallingby and Nancy Barbara, comps.
Lists more than 80 books, booklets, pamphlets, and curricula on sexuality and disability in general as well as on a wide range of specific disabilities. Price and ordering information included for each. *SIECUS (1982), 80 Fifth Ave., Suite 801, New York, N.Y. 10011.*

Sexuality and Physical Disability: Personal Perspectives
David G. Bullard and Susan E. Knight, eds.
Forty-five contributors, many of whom are health professionals who are disabled, discuss personal perspectives and professional issues regarding a wide range of disabilities. Other topics covered are attendant care, body image, parenting, sex education and therapy, and family planning. Highly recommended. *C. V. Mosby (1981), 11830 Westline Industrial Dr., St. Louis, Mo. 63141.*

Who Cares: A Handbook on Sex Education and Counseling Services for Disabled People *Second Edition*
Sex and Disability Project
Unique, outstanding, and comprehensive resource with excellent listings of available services and materials. Highly recommended. *University Park (1982), 300 North Charles St., Baltimore, Md. 21201.*

*

Sexual Abuse of Children

The Best Kept Secret: Sexual Abuse of Children
Florence Rush
Traces historical beginnings of sexual abuse and also includes "a hard look" at discrimination in application of the law governing such abuse. Useful to child-care workers and professionals involved in adult education. *Prentice-Hall (1980), Englewood Cliffs, N.J. 07632.*

Handbook of Clinical Intervention in Child Sexual Abuse
Suzanne M. Sgroi
Discusses a variety of topics that professionals working with sexually abused children face, ranging from reporting, interviewing, and investigating to various forms of therapy that have proven effective. Excellent chapters on developing and evaluating child sexual abuse programs. *Lexington (1982), 125 Spring St., Lexington, Mass. 02173.*

Incest: A Psychological Study of Causes and Effects with Treatment Recommendations
Karen Meiselman
A scholarly study, reported in easy-to-read fashion, of clinical incest cases; includes a comparison of the data obtained with those of previously published studies. *Jossey-Bass (1978), 433 California St., San Francisco, Calif. 94104.*

Physical and Sexual Abuse of Children
David R. Walters
A practical handbook on the subject, including discussion on diagnosis, treatment, and strategies for change. *Indiana University Press (1976), Tenth & Morton, Bloomington, Ind. 47401.*

Sexually Victimized Children
David Finkelhor
An important contribution to the sociological study of sexual victimization and incest. *The Free Press, Macmillan (1979), 866 Third Ave., New York, N.Y. 10022.*

Something Happened to Me
Phyllis E. Sweet
A resource for skilled therapists to use with children who have been sexually abused. Gives children permission to discuss their experiences and feelings. *Mother Courage (1981), 224 State St., Racine, Wis. 53403.*

Sexuality and Religion

Christianity, Social Tolerance, and Homosexuality: Gay People in Western Europe from the Beginning of the Christian Era to the Fourteenth Century
John Boswell
Scholarly analysis of the changes in early Christian attitudes toward homosexuality. Useful for historical background and also for therapists in demonstrating alternatives to Christian mainstream homophobia. *University of Chicago Press (1980), 5801 Ellis Ave., Chicago, Ill. 60637.*

Dimensions of Human Sexuality
Dennis Doherty, ed.
A follow-up volume of critical response to *Human Sexuality: New Directions in American Catholic Thought. Doubleday (1979), 501 Franklin Ave., Garden City, N.Y. 11530.*

Embodiment: An Approach to Sexuality and Christian Thinking
James B. Nelson
Important contribution to ongoing dialogue in the Christian community on the theological meaning of human sexuality. *Pilgrim (1978), 132 West 31st St., New York, N.Y. 10001.*

Homosexuality and Ethics
Edward Batchelor Jr., ed.
Well-chosen, comprehensive selection of essays covering the wide spectrum of Jewish, Protestant, and Roman Catholic views on homosexuality. Useful for reaching a greater understanding of today's issues and debates involving homosexuality. *Pilgrim (1980), 132 West 31st St., New York, N.Y. 10001.*

Human Sexuality: New Directions in American Catholic Thought
Anthony Kosnik, William Carroll, Agnes Cunningham, Ronald Modras, and James Schulte
Prepared by a study group of the Catholic Theological Society of America. Broadens the traditional view of sexuality from "procreative and unitive" to "creative and integrative." While written from the Catholic perspective, its discussions of theological concerns and practical suggestions for pastoral guidance will be of interest to non-Catholics as well. *Paulist (1977), 545 Island Ave., Ramsey, N.J. 07446. Doubleday (1979), 501 Franklin St., Garden City, N.Y. 11530.*

Love, Sex, and Marriage: A Jewish View *New Edition*
Roland B. Gittelsohn
Combined revision of the author's *Consecrated Unto Me* (1965) and its supplement, *Love, Sex, and Marriage* (1976). A textbook for high school students and young adults, with a Jewish viewpoint on all aspects of male/female relationships. *Union of American Hebrew Congregations (1980), 838 Fifth Ave., New York, N.Y. 10021.*

Sex in the World's Religions
Geoffrey Parrinder
Numerous citations from author's sources, stories from his own experiences, along with ample bibliographic suggestions for further study, plus an excellent index make this a very helpful guide to a complicated subject. *Oxford University Press (1980), 200 Madison Ave., New York, N.Y. 10016.*

*

On Pornography

Pornography and Silence: Culture's Revenge Against Nature
Susan Griffin
Author views pornography as a crucial expression of modern culture and a severe contradiction of the basic natural instincts of men and women. Contends that sadomasochism has become endemic in our society. *Harper & Row (1981), 10 East 53rd St., New York, N.Y. 10022.*

Pornography: Men Possessing Women
Andrea Dworkin
Explores the meaning of pornography and the system of power of men over women in which it exists. Presents an impressive array of cogent, angry arguments. *G. P. Putnam's Sons (1981), 200 Madison Ave., New York, N.Y. 10016.*

Take Back the Night: Women on Pornography
Laura Lederer, ed.
A collection of "speak-outs" by women concerned with the increase of violence in pornography. Presents the perspective that pornography is the ideology of a culture that promotes and condones crimes of violence against women. *William Morrow (1980), 105 Madison Ave., New York, N.Y., 10016.*

Women, Sex, and Pornography: A Controversial Study
Beatrice Faust
Author's theory is that when sex is suppressed in the official culture it will surface unofficially in perverse and ugly forms, pointing up the most crucial psychological differences between male and female sexuality. Emphasizes formal sex education programs as a way to understand these differences and therefore ameliorate the pornography problem. *Macmillan (1981), 866 Third Ave., New York, N.Y. 10022.*

*

Special Topics

Circumcision: An American Health Fallacy
Edward Wallerstein
Based on an intensive review of the medical and popular literature, this study challenges the practice of routine circumcision as not only unnecessary and devoid of health benefits, but also potentially harmful and traumatic. *Springer (1980), 200 Park Ave. South, New York, N.Y. 10003.*

Love and Limerence: The Experience of Being in Love
Dorothy Tennov
Around a newly coined term, the author builds a well-documented delineation of the phenomenology of being "head over heels in love." *Stein & Day (1979), Scarborough House, Briarcliff Manor, N.Y. 10510.*

Sex, Crime and the Law
Donal E. J. MacNamara and Edward Sagarin
A survey of the sexual activities illegal in the U.S., discussing legal and sociological definitions, incidence and seriousness, prevailing statutes, research, and recommended reforms. *The Free Press, Macmillan (1978), 866 Third Ave., New York, N.Y. 10022.*

FOR AND ABOUT THE DISABLED

*

General Works

BOOKS AND JOURNALS

Choices: A Sexual Guide for the Physically Handicapped
Maureen Neistadt and Maureen Freda Baker
Makes suggestions for dealing with each of a number of physical problems, such as tremor and loss of mobility, that can result from a wide variety of disabilities and impede sexual functioning. *Massachusetts Rehabilitation Hospital (1979), 125 Nashua St., Boston, Mass. 02114.*

Entitled to Love: The Sexual and Emotional Needs of the Handicapped
Wendy Greengross
Provides direction for professionals in difficult areas such as marriage, residential care, and dealing with parental concerns. Answers the question: What should disabled people learn about sex? *National Marriage Guidance Council (1976). Little Church St., Rugby, England.*

Family Planning Services for Disabled People: A Manual for Service Providers
Ebon Research Systems
Excellent resource that provides guidance for training staff to work with disabled persons, making clinics barrier-free, and offering services related to specific disabilities. Includes a chart of disabling conditions and their effects on reproduction and contraception. *National Clearinghouse for Family Planning Information (1980), P.O. Box 2225, Rockville, Md. 20852.*

Human Sexuality in Health and Illness *Second Edition*
Nancy Fugate Woods
Examines the biophysical nature of human sexuality, sexual health and health care (including preventive and restorative intervention and sexual dysfunction), and clinical aspects of human sexuality in such concerns as chronic illness, paraplegia, and adaptation to changed body image. *C. V. Mosby (1979), 11830 Westline Industrial Dr., St. Louis, Mo. 63141.*

Off Our Backs—Special Issue: Women with Disabilities *Vol. 11, No. 5, May 1981*
A number of the 20 articles are written from a feminist and/or lesbian perspective. Disabilities covered include stroke, visual and hearing impairment, and mastectomy. *Off Our Backs (1981), 1841 Columbia Rd., N.W., Washington, D.C. 20009.*

The Sex and Disability Training Project, 1976–1979: Final Report
David G. Bullard et al.
Report on a nondegree program with trained educator-counselors, most of whom were themselves disabled, to help disabled persons achieve more satisfactory sexual functioning and relationships. *Human Sexuality Program, Dept. of Psychiatry, University of California (1979), 814 Mission St., San Francisco, Calif. 94103.*

Sex and the Handicapped Child
Wendy Greengross
A straightforward, matter-of-fact treatment of the importance of parents' promoting a positive attitude toward their disabled child's sexuality. The author is a disabled woman and a professional sex educator. *National Marriage Guidance Council (n.d.), Little Church St., Rugby, England.*

Sex Education and Counseling of Special Groups: The Mentally and Physically Handicapped, Ill, and Elderly *Second Edition*
Warren R. Johnson and Winifred Kempton
Deals with problem areas in sex education and counseling of handicapped persons and points out danger of losing the individual behind group labels. Offers suggestions for dealing with sex-related topics from masturbation to abortion. *Charles C Thomas (1981), 2600 South First St., Springfield, Ill. 62717.*

Sex, Society, and the Disabled: A Developmental Inquiry into Roles, Reactions, and Responsibilities
Isabel P. Robinault
A chronological discussion of the sexuality of people with physical disabilities. *Harper & Row (1978), 10 East 53rd St., New York, N.Y. 10022.*

Sexual Consequences of Disability
Alex Comfort
Useful collection of articles on a range of disabilities. *Stickley (1978), West Washington Sq., Philadelphia, Pa. 19106.*

Sexual Sabotage: How to Enjoy Sex in Spite of Physical and Emotional Problems
Sherwin A. Kaufman
Written for the general public, this book concerns itself with the sexual repercussions of medical, emotional, and social problems. There is a question-and-answer format covering a wide range of illnesses and other disruptive situations. *Macmillan (1981), 866 Third Ave., New York, N.Y. 10022.*

The Sexual Side of Handicap: A Guide for Caring Professionals
W. F. R. Stewart
An easily readable, handy reference for those beginning to study the sexual world of people with disabilities of various natures. *Woodhead-Faulkner (1979), 8 Market Passage, Cambridge, England.*

Sexuality and Disability
Ami Sha'ked and Susan M. Daniels, eds.
A quarterly journal presenting clinical and research developments in the area of sexuality as they relate to a wide range of physical and mental illnesses and disabling conditions. *Human Sciences, 72 Fifth Ave., New York, N.Y. 10011.*

Sexuality and Physical Disability: Personal Perspectives
David G. Bullard and Susan E. Knight, eds.
Forty-five contributors, many of whom are health professionals who are disabled, discuss personal perspectives and professional issues regarding a wide range of disabilities. Other topics covered are attendant care, body image, parenting, sex education and therapy, and family planning. Highly recommended. *C. V. Mosby (1981), 11830 Westline Industrial Dr., St. Louis, Mo. 63141.*

Sexuality and the Disabled
Michael Barrett and Neville Case, eds.
Proceedings of a workshop held at Royal Ottawa Hospital, April 1976, where most presenters were disabled people. *Sex Information and Education Council of Canada (1976), 423 Castlefield Ave., Toronto, Ontario M5N 1L4, Canada.*

Who Cares? A Handbook on Sex Education and Counseling Services for Disabled People *Second Edition*
Sex and Disability Project
Unique, outstanding, and comprehensive resource with excellent listings of available services and materials. Highly recommended. *University Park (1982), 300 North Charles St., Baltimore, Md. 21201.*

BOOKLETS AND PAMPHLETS

Choices: A Sexual Guide for the Physically Handicapped
Maureen Neistadt and Maureen Freda Baker
Makes suggestions for dealing with each of a number of physical problems, such as tremor and loss of mobility, that can result from a wide variety of disabilities and impede sexual functioning. *Massachusetts Rehabilitation Hospital (1979), 125 Nashua St., Boston, Mass. 02114.*

Essensuals
Designed by and for disabled persons, this is a hand-drawn guide to buying sexual aids. Catalog contains detailed descriptions of uses and misuses of the devices as well as an order form. *Disability and Sensual Horizons (1981), P.O. Box 696, Gracie Station, New York, N.Y. 10028.*

Getting Together
Debra Cornelius, Elaine Makas, and Sophia Chipouras
Tenth in a series on attitudinal barriers facing disabled people, this booklet deals with myths about the sexuality of the disabled and steps that can be taken to overcome them. *RRRI (1981), George Washington University, 603 Park Lane Building, 2025 Eye St., N.W., Washington, D.C. 20052.*

Intimacy and Disability
Barbara F. Waxman and Judi Levin
A comprehensive resource on life skills and sexuality as they relate to the disabled. Growing up, body image, and contraception are discussed at length. An excellent guide for the disabled. *Institute for Information Studies (1982), 200 Little Fall St., Falls Church, Va. 22046.*

Sex Education, Counseling, and Therapy for the Physically Handicapped
American Association of Sex Educators, Counselors, and Therapists
Discusses the impact of eight disabilities on sexuality. *American Association of Sex Educators, Counselors, and Therapists (1979), 11 Dupont Circle, N.W., Washington, D.C. 20036.*

Sex Education for Disabled Persons *Public Affairs Pamphlet #531*
Irving Dickman
The pamphlet alerts professional people working with physically and mentally disabled persons to the importance of providing them with sex education and of helping their parents to do so. *Public Affairs Committee (1975), 381 Park Ave. South, New York, N.Y. 10016.*

Sexual Rights for People Who Happen to Be Handicapped
Sol Gordon and Douglas Bilken
Covers basic concepts of sex information, expression, and birth control services, with a selected list of references. *Ed-U (1979), P.O. Box 583, Fayetteville, N.Y. 13066.*

Toward Intimacy: Family Planning and Sexuality Concerns of Physically Disabled Women
Task Force on the Concerns of Physically Disabled Women
A discussion of various relationships within a disabled woman's life, aimed at promoting communication and understanding. *Human Sciences (1978), 72 Fifth Ave., New York, N.Y. 10011.*

Within Reach: Providing Family Planning Services to Physically Disabled Women
Task Force on Concerns of Physically Disabled Women
Helpful for family planning providers serving disabled women. *Human Sciences (1977), 72 Fifth Ave., New York, N.Y. 10011.*

Xandria Collection: Special Issue for Disabled Persons
Catalog of sexual aids for disabled persons, giving the history of each and advice on how and how not to use them. All items listed are available for purchase through the same distributor. *Lawrence Research Group (1981), Department P.D., P.O. Box 31039, San Francisco, Calif. 94131.*

BIBLIOGRAPHIES

Bibliographies of Holdings of the SIECUS Resource Center and Library: Sexuality and Illness, Disability, or Aging
Leigh Hallingby, comp.
Bibliographies on 30 separate illnesses or disabilities as they relate to sexuality. The 500 unannotated citations include books, chapters from books, periodical articles, booklets, pamphlets, and curricula. Order blank available to those wishing to purchase individual bibliographies. *SIECUS (1980), 80 Fifth Ave., Suite 801, New York, N.Y. 10011.*

Human Sexuality in Physical and Mental Illnesses and Disabilities: An Annotated Bibliography
Ami Sha'ked
Excellent reference tool for all those who provide help with sex-related problems of the ill, aged, and disabled. *Indiana University Press (1979), Tenth & Morton, Bloomington, Ind. 47405.*

Sex and Disability: A Resource Guide to Books, Pamphlets, Articles and Audio, Visual, and Tactile Materials
Eleanor Smith, Paula Silver, and Katrine Hughes
An easy-to-read bibliography with annotations and comments on the helpfulness of each entry. Very usefully laid out. *A Central Place (1981), 477 15th St., Oakland, Calif. 94612.*

Sex and Disability: A Selected Bibliography
M. G. Eisenberg
Contains hundreds of references to literature published from 1942–1978, with 80 percent from 1960 on. Very useful for a wide range of disabilities. *Rehabilitation Psychology (1978), Box 26034, Tempe, Ariz. 85282.*

Sexuality and Disability: A Bibliography of Resources Available for Purchase
Leigh Hallingby and Nancy Barbara, comps.
Lists more than 80 books, booklets, pamphlets, and curricula on sexuality and disability in general as well as on a wide range of specific disabilities. Price and ordering information included for each. *SIECUS (1982), 80 Fifth Ave., Suite 801, New York, N.Y. 10011.*

Sexuality and Disability: A Selected Annotated Bibliography
Debra Cornelius, Elaine Makas, and Sophia Chipouras
Product of literature searches conducted by the Sex and Disability Project, containing over 400 listings. *RRRI (1979), George Washington University, 603 Park Lane Building, 2025 Eye St., N.W., Washington, D.C. 20052.*

Sexuality and the Disabled: An Annotated Bibliography
Includes 200 citations to books, periodical articles, curricula, conference papers, and dissertations. *Katharine Dexter McCormick Library (1981), Planned Parenthood Federation of America, 810 Seventh Ave., New York, N.Y. 10019.*

CURRICULUM

Sexuality and Sexual Assault: Disabled Perspectives
Charles K. Stuart and Virginia Stuart
Curriculum guide for development of workshop for professionals on incest, rape, and sexual abuse of disabled people. Highly recommended. *Charles K. Stuart, Director of Counseling Services (1980), Southwest State University, Marshall, Minn. 56258.*

Cancer

Body Image, Self-Esteem, and Sexuality in Cancer Patients
J. M. Vaeth, R. C. Blomberg, and L. Adler, eds.
The conference on which this outstanding book is based was a first in the specific area of cancer and its possible effects on sexuality and self-esteem in patients of all ages. *S. Karger (1980), 150 Fifth Ave., Suite 1105, New York, N.Y. 10011.*

Sexual Rehabilitation of the Urologic Cancer Patient
Andrew C. von Eschenbach and Dorothy Rodriguez, eds.
This collection of articles is derived from papers presented at a 1979 seminar at the University of Texas in Houston. A valuable book for any individual involved in the total care of patients with urologic cancer. *G. K. Hall (1981), 70 Lincoln St., Boston, Mass. 02111.*

Sexuality and Cancer
Jean M. Stoklosa, David C. Bullard, Ernest H. Rosenbaum, and Isadora D. Rosenbaum
Sensitively written discussion with useful sections on ostomy, laryngectomy, and mastectomy. *Bull (1980), Box 208, Palo Alto, Calif. 94302.*

*

Cerebral Palsy

Cerebral Palsy and Sexuality
Nathan Liskey and Phillip Stephens
A collection of case studies focusing particularly on sexual development and adult sexual expression. *Disabled Students on Campus Organization (1978), California State University, c/o Handicapped Students Services, Fresno, Calif. 93740.*

Sex for the Handicapped Man: An Educational Booklet
Weldon Leon Sutton
An illustrated, self-help manual written at a sixth-grade reading level, printed in large type, and tabbed for easy reference. Although the drawings are oriented toward people with cerebral palsy, the text is applicable for the disabled in general. Chapter titles include: "How to Relax," "Masturbation," "Foreplay," and "Ask Questions." *Self-Help Manual (1981), 8595 Conway Dr., Riverside, Calif. 92504.*

*

Hearing Impaired

Sexuality and Deafness
Robert R. Davila, Della Fitz-Gerald, Max Fitz-Gerald, and Clarence M. Williams
A compilation of eight articles. Deals primarily with the need for instruction in

sexuality for hearing-impaired persons of all ages. *Gallaudet College, Outreach Services, Pre-College Programs (1979), MSSD Box 114F Kendall Green, Washington, D.C. 20002.*

Signs for Sexuality: A Resource Manual
Susan D. Doughten, Marlyn B. Minkin, and Laurie E. Rosen
Contains more than 600 photographs illustrating 300 signed words and phrases associated with human sexuality. Bound to lie flat, leaving hands free for communication. *Planned Parenthood of Seattle/King County (1978), 2211 East Madison, Seattle, Wash. 98112.*

Signs of Sexual Behavior
James Woodward
Each sign, along with its etymology, is explained. Author also discusses deaf culture as it relates to the ever-changing signs. *T. J. (1979), 817 Silver Spring Ave., Suite 305D, Silver Spring, Md. 20910.*

*

Mentally Handicapped

BOOKS AND BOOKLETS

Developing Community Acceptance of Sex Education for the Mentally Retarded
Medora Bass
Outlines a program of two or three meetings for parents or staff to explain the need for sex education and to indicate concepts to be taught to the mentally handicapped. *SIECUS (1972), 80 Fifth Ave., Suite 801, New York, N.Y. 10011.*

An Easy Guide to Loving Carefully for Men and Women
Lyn McKee, Winifred Kempton, and Lynne Stiggall
Basic information about sexual anatomy, reproduction, and contraception, presented in large print with many illustrations. Suitable for higher functioning mentally handicapped people to read on their own or with a parent or professional. *Planned Parenthood of Contra Costa (1980), 1291 Oakland Blvd., Walnut Creek, Calif. 94596.*

Handicapped Married Couples
Ann Craft and Michael Craft
Gives an account of authors' research of a sample of 25 marriages with at least one mentally handicapped spouse. Suggests ways in which service to such couples might be improved and provides materials for teaching purposes. *Routledge and Kegan Paul (1979), 9 Park St., Boston, Mass. 02108.*

Human Sexuality and the Mentally Retarded
Felix F. de la Cruz and Gerald D. Laveck, eds.
Examines physical and psychological aspects of sexual behavior, relating them to the needs of those with learning handicaps. *Brunner/Mazel (1973), 19 Union Sq. West, New York, N.Y. 10003.*

Like Normal People
Robert Meyers
Warm, touching story of the marriage of Roger Meyers and Virginia Hensler, written by Roger's brother. Describes long struggle of these two mentally handicapped individuals to lead a dignified life. *McGraw-Hill (1978), 1221 Avenue of the Americas, New York, N.Y. 10020.*

Organizing Community Resources in Sexuality, Counseling, and Family Planning for the Retarded: A Community Worker's Manual
Karin Rolett
Self-instructional format moves reader step by step toward organizing informational or service programs. *Carolina Population Center (1976), University of North Carolina, University Sq., Chapel Hill, N.C. 27514.*

Sex and the Mentally Handicapped
Michael Craft and Ann Craft
Written for professionals and parents caring for the mentally handicapped, this British book looks at many of the questions, anxieties, and fears raised by the sexuality of this group. Offers guidelines to those wishing to plan sex education programs. *Routledge and Kegan Paul (1978), 9 Park St., Boston, Mass. 02108.*

Sex Education for Persons with Disabilities That Hinder Learning: A Teacher's Guide
Winifred Kempton
Invaluable resource for instructors on human sexuality for students with learning problems, stressing the need to integrate sexuality with every facet of human experience. *Planned Parenthood of Southeastern Pennsylvania (1975), 1220 Sansom St., Philadelphia, Pa. 19107.*

Sexual Rights and Responsibilities of the Mentally Retarded
Medora S. Bass, ed.
Comes to grips with social attitudes and educational policy relating to the sexual rights of the retarded. *Medora S. Bass (1975), 1387 East Valley Rd., Santa Barbara, Calif. 93108.*

CURRICULA AND TESTS

Becoming Me: A Personal Adjustment Guide for Secondary Students
Theresa Throckmorton
For use with secondary special education students. Focuses on functional living skills such as decision making, problem solving, and sexual and social fulfillment.

A content outline, behavioral objectives, suggested resources, and learning activities are included for each topic covered. *Grand Rapids Public Schools (1980), 143 Bostwick, N.E., Grand Rapids, Mich. 49503.*

Being Me: A Social/Sexual Training Guide for Those Who Work with the Developmentally Disabled
Jean Edwards and Suzan Wapnick
A curriculum for teachers working with developmentally disabled individuals from first grade through middle age. Can be used with severely or more mildly handicapped children or adults. *Ednick Communications (1981), Box 3612, Portland, Ore. 97208.*

Education for Adulthood
Madeline Greenbaum and Sandra Noll
Contains two sections: a training guide for those who will teach the curriculum and a curriculum for mentally retarded adolescents and adults who need a better understanding of social and sexual life. Includes units on body image, feelings, acceptance of disability, expressing sexuality, and interpersonal relationships. *Staten Island Mental Health Society (1982), Center for Developmental Disabilities, 657 Castleton Ave., Staten Island, N.Y. 10301.*

Essential Adult Sex Education (EASE) Curriculum
David Zelman
Includes curriculum guide, pre- and post-tests, birth control and menstruation kit, and profile sheets. Highly regarded for its comprehensiveness and ease of use. *SFA, James Stanfield Film Associates (1979), P.O. Box 1983, Santa Monica, Calif. 90406.*

Feeling Good About Yourself: A Guide for People Working with People Who Have Disabilities *Second Edition*
Gloria Blum and Barry Blum
This curriculum guide for teaching sex education in the special education classroom is now available in a new, expanded edition. In addition to socialization and decision-making skills, a wide variety of sexual topics is covered. The continuing focus is on self-esteem as the essential ingredient in preparation for adulthood. *Feeling Good Associates (1981), 507 Palma Way, Mill Valley, Calif. 94941.*

A Guide for Teaching Human Sexuality to the Mentally Handicapped *Third Edition*
Phyllis Cooksey and Pamela Brown
This curriculum guide contains nine categories such as contraception and interpersonal relations. Under each are listed topics to cover, points to make, and suggested activities and resources. A simple but very practical approach to teaching the mentally handicapped about sexuality. *Planned Parenthood of Minnesota (1981), 1965 Ford Pkwy., St. Paul, Minn. 55116.*

Guidelines for Training in Sexuality and the Mentally Handicapped
Winifred Kempton and Rose Forman
Not a textbook, but a proposed training program for those working with staff, aides, or parents involved with the mentally handicapped. *Planned Parenthood of Southeastern Pennsylvania (1976), 1220 Sansom St., Philadelphia, Pa. 19107.*

Human Sexuality: A Portfolio for the Mentally Retarded
Victoria Livingston and Mary E. Knapp
Consists of 10 separate drawings on stiffened paper, with discussion suggestions for the teacher printed on the back of each plate. Content areas include male and female genitalia, girl to woman, boy to man, masturbation, and sexual intercourse. *Planned Parenthood of Seattle–King County (1974), 2211 East Madison, Seattle, Wash. 98112.*

Lincoln School: Human Growth and Development
William W. Krate et al.
A curriculum guide oriented toward trainable mentally impaired people from age two through adulthood. Includes suggestions on parental involvement, staff development, assessment and evaluation, and four comprehensive curricular units: self-concept, health and self-care, human growth, and social developments. *Lincoln School HGD (1980), 860 Crahen Rd., N.E., Grand Rapids, Mich. 49506.*

Personal Development and Sexuality: A Curriculum Guide for Developmentally Disabled
Provides instructional content and many excellent group activities in areas of sex education and skill development. A fine resource for those working with the mentally handicapped. *Planned Parenthood of Pierce County (1978), 312 Broadway Terrace Building, Tacoma, Wash. 98402.*

A Resource Guide in Sex Education for the Mentally Retarded
SIECUS and American Alliance for Health, Physical Education & Recreation
Concepts to be taught are outlined, followed by comments, content, and activities relating to each. *SIECUS (1971), 80 Fifth Ave., Suite 801, New York, N.Y. 10011.*

Sexuality and Social Awareness: A Curriculum for Moderately Autistic and/or Neurologically Impaired Individuals
Dawn A. Lieberman and Mary Bonyai Melone
Extremely valuable for sex educators working with lower functioning mentally handicapped individuals. *Benhaven (1979), 9 Saint Ronan Terr., New Haven, Conn. 06511.*

Socio-Sexual Knowledge and Attitude Test (SSKAT)
Joel R. Wish, Katherine Fiechtl McCombs, and Barbara Edmonson
Can be used with mentally retarded persons and others whose language is limited. Responses to most questions consist of the subject's pointing to a choice of pictures and indicating "yes" or "no." There are 13 subtests, which can determine both sex

knowledge and attitudes. Manual presents data from use of SSKAT with 200 retarded adults ranging in age from 18 to 42. *Stoelting (1976), 1350 South Koster Ave., Chicago, Ill. 60623.*

Special Education Curriculum on Sexual Exploitation
Developmental Disabilities Project of Seattle Rape Relief
Designed for teaching mentally and physically handicapped students to be aware of sexual exploitation and to protect themselves. Two self-contained kits (elementary and secondary levels) provide materials such as teacher's guide, body maps, slides, tapes, and 20 pamphlets to be given to parents. *Comprehensive Health Education Foundation (1981), 20814 Pacific Hwy. South, Seattle, Wash. 98188.*

Teaching Sex Education to Adults Who Are Labeled Mentally Retarded
Al Strauss
Deals with self-appreciation, friendship, and love, as well as anatomy, physiology, and birth control. *Al Strauss (1976), P.O. Box 2141, Oshkosh, Wis. 54903.*

PARENT GUIDES

An Easy Guide for Caring Parents: Sexuality and Socialization—A Book for Parents of People with Mental Handicaps
Lyn McKee and Virginia Blacklidge
An honest, upbeat book about the social and sexual needs of people with mental handicaps. Valuable aid to both parents and educators. *Planned Parenthood of Contra Costa (1981), 1291 Oakland Blvd., Walnut Creek, Calif. 94596.*

Love, Sex, and Birth Control for the Mentally Retarded: A Guide for Parents
Winifred Kempton, Medora Bass, and Sol Gordon
Thoughtful guide covering sex education and sexual responsibility. Spanish edition also available. *Planned Parenthood of Southeastern Pennsylvania (1973), 1220 Sansom St., Philadelphia, Pa. 19107.*

Sara and Allen: The Right to Choose *Revised Edition*
Jean Edwards
Written for parents who want to begin to deal openly with the social/sexual needs of their retarded children. Encouraging, informal, practical tone. *Ednick Communications (1980), P.O. Box 3612, Portland, Ore. 97208.*

*

Multiple Sclerosis

Guide to Program Planning on Sexuality and Multiple Sclerosis
Ann Barrett and Michael Barrett
Includes well-devised exercises for groups dealing with sexuality and multiple sclerosis. *Multiple Sclerosis Society of Canada (1978), 130 Bloor St. West, Toronto, Ontario M5S 1N5, Canada.*

Sexuality and Multiple Sclerosis *Revised Edition*
Michael Barrett
Useful booklet for people with multiple sclerosis and professionals working with them. *Multiple Sclerosis Society of Canada (1982), 130 Bloor St. West, Toronto, Ontario M5Ś 1N5, Canada.*

Ostomy

Pregnancy and the Woman with an Ostomy
Sex and the Female Ostomate
Sex and the Male Ostomate
Sex, Courtship, and the Single Ostomate
Well-written booklets for ostomates and those working with them.*United Ostomy Association (1973), 2001 West Beverly Blvd., Los Angeles, Calif. 90057.*

Sexual Counseling for Ostomates
Ellen A. Shipes and Sally T. Lehr
A commonsense approach to sexual counseling of ostomates, covering easy-to-understand techniques. *Charles C Thomas (1980), 2600 South First St., Springfield, Ill. 62717.*

Spinal Cord Injured

Female Sexuality Following Spinal Cord Injury
Elle Friedman Becker
Offers an opportunity to understand the struggle of a quadriplegic or paraplegic woman in a world that represses and defines her sexual expression and identity, and to learn what disabled people look for from the professional community, their family, and friends. *Cheever (1978), P.O. Box 700, Bloomington, Ill. 61701.*

A Handbook on Sexuality After Spinal Cord Injury
Joanne M. Taggie and M. Scott Manley
A workbook to help spinal cord injured people and their partners identify and begin to work out their feelings as sexual individuals. *M. Scott Manley (1978), 3425 South Clarkson, Englewood, Colo. 80110.*

Human Sexuality and Rehabilitation Medicine: Sexual Functioning Following Spinal Cord Injury
Ami Sha'ked, ed.
Fifteen chapters for health-care professionals who deal with spinal cord injury as well as other disabilities, to help people adjust to their problems. *Williams and Wilkins (1981), 428 East Preston St., Baltimore, Md. 21202.*

Psychological, Sexual, Social, and Vocational Aspects of Spinal Cord Injury: A Selected Bibliography
Gary T. Athelstan et al.
Unannotated bibliography containing almost 900 citations, of which more than 200 fall under the heading "Sexual Aspects." *Rehabilitation Psychology(1978), Box 26034, Tempe, Ariz. 85282.*

The Sensuous Wheeler: Sexual Adjustment for the Spinal Cord Injured
Barry J. Rabin
Informal, positive treatment of the subject, stressing the sharing of sexual responsibilities and vulnerabilities. *Multi Media Resource Center (1980), 1525 Franklin St., San Francisco, Calif. 94109.*

Sex and the Spinal Cord Injured: Some Questions and Answers
M. G. Eisenberg and L. C. Rustad
Questions discussed include areas such as physical attractiveness, aging, drugs, catheters, divorce, adoption, and alternative methods of sexual expression. *Superintendent of Documents, U.S. Government Printing Office (1975), Washington, D.C. 20402.*

Sexual Options for Paraplegics and Quadriplegics
Thomas O. Mooney, Theodore M. Cole, and Richard A. Chilgren
Because the senior author is a near quadriplegic himself, a personalized style of writing results that, with the explicit photographs, provides an excellent self-help teaching or counseling resource. *Little, Brown (1975), 34 Beacon St., Boston, Mass. 02106.*

Sexuality and the Spinal Cord Injured Woman
Sue Bregman
Booklet providing guidelines concerning social and sexual adjustment for spinal cord injured women and health professionals who work with them. *Sister Kenny Institute (1975), Dept. 199, 800 East 28th St. at Chicago Ave., Minneapolis, Minn. 55407.*

*

Visually Impaired

Sex Education and Family Life for Visually Handicapped Children and Youth: A Resource Guide
Irving R. Dickman et al.
Grew out of project sponsored by SIECUS and American Foundation for the Blind. Most useful for its developmental sequence of concepts to be taught and learning activities. *SIECUS (1975), 80 Fifth Ave., Suite 801, New York, N.Y. 10011.*

Sex Education for the Visually Handicapped in Schools and Agencies: Selected Papers
Sound advice on the development and implementation of sex education programs for the visually impaired, from professionals in a variety of settings. *American Foundation for the Blind (1975), 15 West 16th St., New York, N.Y. 10011.*

BRAILLE & LARGE-PRINT PAMPHLETS

Birth Control: All the Methods That Work and the Ones That Don't
Planned Parenthood of New York City
Special editions of a well-known publication. *Braille edition: Iowa Commission for the Blind (1977), 4th and Keosauqua Way, Des Moines, Iowa 50309. Large-type edition: Foundation for Blind Children (1977), 1201 North 85th Pl., Scottsdale, Ariz. 85257.*

Braille Pamphlets
Pamphlets (a number of which are braille versions of widely used materials) are available on the following topics: sexually transmitted diseases, birth control, menstruation, sex information for teenagers, sex education in the home, issues in sexuality for disabled persons, DES, and breast self-examination. *Planned Parenthood of Humboldt County, 2316 Harrison, Eureka, Calif. 95501.*

For Boys: A Book About Girls
Braille booklet explaining menstruation. Includes braille diagrams of female reproductive system. *Personal Products (1980), Milltown, N.J. 08850.*

Growing Up and Liking It
Booklet explaining menstruation to girls, available in braille. *Personal Products (1980), Milltown, N.J. 08850.*

Large Print Materials
Eleven separate pamphlets covering birth control pills, intrauterine devices, diaphragms, condoms, and other contraceptive topics. *A Central Place (1981), 477 15th St., Oakland, Calif. 94612.*

*

Other Disabilities

Living and Loving with Arthritis
Jo-An Boggs
Reassuring booklet on sexual adjustment for persons with arthritis. *Arthritis Center of Hawaii (1978), 347 North Kuakini St., Honolulu, Hawaii 96817.*

Sex and Dialysis
Barbara Ulery
A valuable resource in this special area of concern. *Barbara Ulery (1979), P.O. Box 462, Durango, Colo. 81301.*

Sex and Spina Bifida
W. F. R. Stewart
Consumer-oriented booklet covering effects of spina bifida on growing up, anatomy, birth control, and sexual functioning. *Tavistock House North (1978), Tavistock Sq., London, England.*

Sex Education for Deaf-Blind Children: Workshop Proceedings
Carmella Ficociello, ed.
Proceedings of a 1976 conference. *International Research Institute (1976), P.O. Box 3318, Austin, Texas 78764.*

Sexuality and Neuromuscular Disease
Frances Anderson, Joan Bardach, and Joseph Goodgold
This monograph's recommendations for helping disabled individuals with neuromuscular disease achieve sexual fulfillment are derived from interviews with patients, their families, and physical therapists as well as from literature surveys. *Institute of Rehabilitation Medicine (1979), New York University Medical Center, 400 East 34th St., New York, N.Y. 10016.*

So Desperate the Fight: An Innovative Approach to Chronic Illness
Warren R. Johnson
Dr. Johnson, a well-known writer on the subject of sexuality and disability, depicts poignantly his struggles and triumphs in evolving and practicing a philosophy for dealing with the debilitating disease of scleroderma. *Institute for Rational Living (1981), 45 East 65th St., New York, N.Y. 10021.*

Sound Sex and the Aging Heart
Lee Dreisinger Scheingold and Nathaniel N. Wagner
Discusses sex in the middle and later years, with special reference to cardiac problems. *Human Sciences (1974), 72 Fifth Ave., New York, N.Y. 10011.*

FOR GENERAL READERS

*

Young Children

Did the Sun Shine Before You Were Born?
Sol and Judith Gordon
A book that parents can read with their children, ages 3 to 6. In addition to answering the question "Where do babies come from?" clearly and directly, it deals with other aspects of how different kinds of families live and grow. *Ed-U (1977), P.O. Box 583, Fayetteville, N.Y. 13066.*

Girls Are Girls and Boys Are Boys—So What's the Difference? *Revised Edition*
Sol Gordon
A nonsexist, liberating sex education book for children. *Ed-U (1979), P.O. Box 583, Fayetteville, N.Y. 13066.*

Growing Up Feeling Good: A Child's Introduction to Sexuality
Stephanie Waxman
An excellent introduction to many important concepts about human sexuality, presented with simplicity and dignity. *Panjandrum (1979), 11321 Iowa Ave., Los Angeles, Calif. 90025.*

How Babies Are Made
Andrew C. Andry and Steve Schepp
The story of reproduction in plants, animals, and humans, told through the use of color photographs of paper sculptures. Factually accurate and simple enough to be understood by the youngest group. *Time-Life (1974), 777 Duke St., Alexandria, Va. 22314.*

How Was I Born?
Lennart Nilsson
To be read by parents with their children. Tells the story of reproduction and birth using a combination of the famous Nilsson photographs of fetal development with warm family scenes and other illustrations. *Delacorte (1975), 1 Dag Hammarskjold Plaza, New York, N.Y. 10017.*

Our New Baby: A Picture Story About Birth for Parents and Children
Grethe Fagerstrom and Gunilla Hansson
Translated from the Swedish edition, this book is the story of a year in the life of a family going through the range of emotions—happiness, anger, jealousy, and solidarity—that all families experience. During the year a new baby arrives, and the parents and children discuss how she was conceived, developed, and born, and what she means to the family. *Barron's Educational Series (1982), 113 Crossways Park Dr., Woodbury, N.Y. 11797.*

What Is a Girl? What Is a Boy?
Stephanie Waxman
A simply written, nonsexist message for young children: names, hair lengths, interests, clothing, and emotions do not identify a person as a boy or a girl—only a person's genitals can do that. *Peace (1976), 3828 Willat Ave., Culver City, Calif. 90230.*

"Where Did I Come From?"
Peter Mayle
The facts of life without any nonsense, with illustrations and humor. *Lyle Stuart (1973), 120 Enterprise Ave., Secaucus, N.J. 07094.*

X: A Fabulous Child's Story
Lois Gould
Entertaining, imaginatively presented story about what it means to be male or female. Fun for the whole family. *Daughters (1978), Ms590, Box 42999, Houston, Texas 77042. Grosset & Dunlap (1980), 51 Madison Ave., New York, N.Y. 10010.*

*

Preteens

Love and Sex and Growing Up
Corinne B. Johnson and Eric W. Johnson
Covers a broad range of topics to help preadolescents think about what being a man or a woman means in today's world. *Bantam (1979), 666 Fifth Ave., New York, N.Y. 10019.*

Period
Joann Gardner-Loulan, Bonnie Lopez, and Marcia Quackenbush
Reassuring, cleverly illustrated book about menstruation, explaining why all girls are normal at the same time that everyone is special. Includes personal narratives. Spanish edition, entitled *Periodo*, also available. *Volcano (1979), 330 Ellis St., San Francisco, Calif. 94102.*

"What's Happening to Me?"
Peter Mayle
A clear, concise, straightforward guide to puberty for preadolescent children. *Lyle Stuart (1975), 120 Enterprise Ave., Secaucus, N.J. 07094.*

Early Teens

Boys and Sex
Girls and Sex *Revised Editions*
Wardell B. Pomeroy
These classic sexual guides for teenage boys and girls have now been updated. *Delacorte (1981), 1 Dag Hammarskjold Plaza, New York, N.Y. 10017.*

Changes: You and Your Body
CHOICE
Easy-to-read booklet about puberty, prepared with input from a panel of teenagers. Highly recommended. Available in Spanish. *CHOICE (1978), 1501 Cherry St., Philadelphia, Pa. 19102.*

Facts About Sex for Today's Youth *Revised Edition*
Sol Gordon
A short, direct approach in explaining anatomy, reproduction, love, and sex problems. Includes slang terms when giving definitions, and a section answering the 10 questions most frequently asked. Well illustrated. *Ed-U (1979), P.O. Box 583, Fayetteville, N.Y. 13066.*

Facts About VD for Today's Youth *Revised Edition*
Sol Gordon
Up-to-date, accurate information written in clear and simple language. Stresses prevention *Ed-U (1979), P.O. Box 583, Fayetteville, N.Y. 13066.*

Love and Sex in Plain Language *Revised Edition*
Eric W. Johnson
Provides basic information on sexuality. Emphasizes that sexuality should always be seen in the context of one's total personality and expressed in responsible, respectful interpersonal relationships. *Bantam (1979), 666 Fifth Ave., New York, N.Y. 10019*

Sex: Telling It Straight
Eric W. Johnson
A simple but honest treatment of those topics in human sexuality of greatest concern to adolescents. Written for teenage slow readers, especially those within problem environments, and presents positive views on sex without preaching or moralizing. *Harper & Row (1979), 10 East 53rd St., New York, N.Y. 10022.*

Sex with Love: A Guide for Young People
Eleanor Hamilton
Includes discussion of the rituals of early dating and fulfilling the body's need for affection and sexual expression. *Beacon (1978), 25 Beacon St., Boston, Mass. 02108.*

What Teens Want to Know but Don't Know How to Ask
A concise pamphlet that answers the questions most adolescents ask about sex. *Planned Parenthood Federation of America (1976), 810 Seventh Ave., New York, N.Y. 10019.*

*

Late Teens

Am I Parent Material?
A pamphlet listing thoughtful questions about an important decision. Available in Spanish. *National Alliance for Optional Parenthood (1977), 1439 Rhode Island Ave., N.W., Washington, D.C. 20005.*

Changes: Becoming a Teenage Parent
Krail Brooks and Rose DeWolf
Excellent booklet for single pregnant teenagers, providing information on such topics as prenatal care, birth, emotional changes, finances, possible living arrangements, and adjustment to motherhood. Attractively presented. *Planned Parenthood of Southeastern Pennsylvania (1979), 1220 Sansom St., Philadelphia, Pa. 19107.*

Changing Bodies, Changing Lives
Ruth Bell and other co-authors of Our Bodies, Ourselves
A forthright, nonjudgmental book for teens that confronts their real concerns about sex and relationships. Highly recommended. *Random House (1980), 201 East 50th St., New York, N.Y. 10022.*

The Facts of Love: Living, Loving, and Growing Up
Alex Comfort and Jane Comfort
A dynamic book about sexuality, ideal as a catalyst for conversations with young people. *Crown (1980), 1 Park Ave., New York, N.Y. 10016.*

Growing Up Sexual
Eleanor Morrison, Kay Starks, Cynda Hyndman, and Nina Ronzio
Unique view of patterns of human sexual development based on anonymous autobiographical papers by students in a college human sexuality course. Also recommended for parents. *Brooks/Cole (1980), Monterey, Calif. 93940.*

Learning About Sex: A Contemporary Guide for Young Adults
Gary F. Kelly
Without neglecting basic factual information, focuses on attitudes and the process of sexual decision making. Highly recommended. *Barron's Educational Series (1977), 113 Crossways Park Dr., Woodbury, N.Y. 11797.*

Parenting: A Guide for Young People
Sol Gordon and Mina Wollin
A thoroughly modern exposition to prepare potential parents for mature parenting roles. *William H. Sadlier (1975), 11 Park Pl., New York, N.Y. 10007.*

Sex and Birth Control: A Guide for the Young *Revised Edition*
E. James Lieberman and Ellen Peck
Written to encourage sensible and responsible use of birth control and to encourage young people to develop principles and values by which they will live their sexual lives. *Harper & Row (1981), 10 East 53rd St., New York, N.Y. 10022.*

Sex Education for Adolescents: A Bibliography of Low-Cost Materials
Criteria used for selection: appropriateness to adolescents in readability; cost of $6.00 or less; and values perspective responsibly represented in contemporary terms but without limitation as to position on the conservative-liberal spectrum. *American Library Association (1980), Order Department, 50 East Huron St., Chicago, Ill. 60611.*

Sexuality: Decisions, Attitudes, Relationships
Booklet dealing with how to clarify feelings about sexuality and relationships. *Planned Parenthood of Southeastern Pennsylvania (1979), 1220 Sansom St., Philadelphia, Pa. 19107.*

The Teenage Body Book
Kathy McCoy and Charles Wibbelsman
A thoughtfully written, reassuring resource for adolescents, dealing with their various psychological and physiological concerns. *Pocket Books, Simon & Schuster, (1979) 1230 Avenue of the Americas, New York, N.Y. 10020.*

A Way of Love, A Way of Life: A Young Person's Introduction to What It Means to Be Gay
Frances Hanckel and John Cunningham
A unique, sensitive book written by people who are *having* the experience for people who want to *understand* it. *Lothrop, Lee & Shepard (1979), 105 Madison Ave., New York, N.Y. 10016.*

Why Am I So Miserable If These Are the Best Years of My Life? *Revised Edition*
Andrea Boroff Eagan
Encourages young women to be self-determining. Includes factual information on physiology, menstruation, sexually transmitted diseases, and birth control. *Avon (1979), 959 Eighth Ave., New York, N.Y. 10019.*

Your Sexual Freedom: Letters to Students
Richard Hettlinger
Addressed to young people who are expected to be liberated and informed in regard to sexuality but who in fact, must cope with a variety of difficulties.

Encourages them to develop their own distinctive sexual selves. *Continuum (1982), 575 Lexington Ave., New York, N.Y. 10022.*

*

Adults

FOR MEN

Good Sex: A Healthy Man's Guide to Sexual Fulfillment
Gary F. Kelly
Insightful and sensitive self-help book for men who want more total sexual fulfillment. *Harcourt Brace Jovanovich (1979), 757 Third Ave., New York, N.Y. 10017. New American Library, 1633 Broadway, New York, N.Y. 10019.*

The Hite Report on Male Sexuality
Shere Hite
Depicts the enormous variety and diversity of male sexuality expressions and attitudes and presents provocative ideas about the nature of sexual intercourse and other forms of sexual behavior. *Alfred A. Knopf (1981), 201 East 50th St., New York, N.Y. 10022.*

Lifelong Sexual Vigor: How to Avoid and Overcome Impotence
Marvin B. Brooks and Sally West Brooks
A definitive work and comprehensive review on the subject of erectile dysfunction, presented in fluid prose style. *Doubleday (1981), 501 Franklin Ave., Garden City, N.Y. 11530.*

Male "Menopause": Crisis in the Middle Years *Public Affairs Pamphlet #526*
Theodore Irwin
Useful pamphlet on the subject. *Public Affairs Committee (1975), 381 Park Ave. South, New York, N.Y. 10016.*

Male Sexuality
Bernie Zilbergeld
For the man who wants to get more in touch with his own sexuality or for any woman who wants to understand more fully the potentials of male sexuality. *Little, Brown (1978), 34 Beacon St., Boston, Mass. 02106. Bantam, 666 Fifth Ave., New York, N.Y. 10019.*

Man's Body: An Owner's Manual
The Diagram Group
Clear answers to questions about how the male body functions, from infancy to old age. *Bantam (1976), 666 Fifth Ave., New York, N.Y. 10019.*

Men in Love
Nancy Friday
Based on 3000 responses, explores men's sexual fantasies within a theoretical framework, which gives a basis for analyzation and interpretation. *Delacorte (1980), 1 Dag Hammarskjold Plaza, New York, N.Y. 10017.*

Men's Bodies, Men's Selves
Sam Julty
A comprehensive collection of thoughts and information relating to men and masculinity in contemporary society. *Delta, Dell (1979), 1 Dag Hammarskjold Plaza, New York, N.Y. 10017.*

Sexual Solutions: An Informative Guide
Michael Castleman
Using a nonclinical approach, the author gives readers an effective framework of information for studying and reshaping their perception of men as sexual beings. *Simon & Schuster (1980), 1230 Avenue of the Americas, New York, N.Y. 10020.*

Women: A Book for Men
James Wagenvoord and Peyton Bailey, eds.
With its companion book, *Men: A Book for Women*, recommended for joint reading by heterosexual couples needing or wanting to deepen their understanding of each other as sexual persons. *Avon (1979), 959 Eighth Ave., New York, N.Y. 10019.*

FOR WOMEN

Becoming Orgasmic: A Sexual Growth Program for Women
Julia Heiman, Leslie LoPiccolo, and Joseph LoPiccolo
A detailed growth program for women who feel they have problems in experiencing orgasm. Also includes a section relating to male partners. The emphasis is on orgasm as a part, rather than the only or primary goal, of sexuality and sexual experience. *Prentice-Hall (1976), Englewood Cliffs, N.J. 07632.*

For Each Other: Sharing Sexual Intimacy
Lonnie Barbach
Anchor, Doubleday (1982), 501 Franklin Ave., Garden City, N.Y. 11530.

For Yourself: The Fulfillment of Female Sexuality
Lonnie Barbach
Written primarily for women having difficulty achieving orgasm. Discusses sources of confusion about female sexuality, describes female sexual physiology, and suggests specific exercises women can do at home. *Doubleday (1976), 501 Franklin Ave., Garden City, N.Y. 11530. New American Library, 1633 Broadway, New York, N.Y. 10019.*

The Hite Report
Shere Hite
Based on responses to in-depth questionnaires returned by some 3000 women. A provocative and revealing study that examines the subject of female sexuality from the inside. Makes extensive use of direct quotes. *Macmillan (1976), 866 Third Ave., New York, N.Y. 10022. Dell, 1 Dag Hammarskjold Plaza, New York, N.Y. 10017.*

The Joy of Lesbian Sex
Emily L. Sisley and Bertha Harris
A–Z format. First major sex manual for lesbians, discussing their needs and concerns. *Crown (1977), 1 Park Ave., New York, N.Y. 10016.*

Men: A Book for Women
James Wagenvoord and Peyton Bailey, eds.
With its companion book, *Women: A Book for Men*, recommended for joint reading by heterosexual couples needing or wanting to deepen their understanding of each other as sexual persons. *Avon (1978), 959 Eighth Ave., New York, N.Y. 10019.*

The Menopause Book
Louisa Rose, ed.
A carefully documented, highly readable compilation of information aimed at dispelling myths surrounding sexuality and aging. Raises some important issues concerning men and women in the middle period. *Hawthorn (1977), 2 Park Ave., New York, N.Y. 10016.*

A New View of a Woman's Body: A Fully Illustrated Guide
Federation of Feminist Women's Health Centers
A feminist perspective on female sexuality written by pioneers in the women's self-help movement. Discussion and drawings of the clitoris are particularly notable. *Simon & Schuster (1981), 1230 Avenue of the Americas, New York, N.Y.10020.*

Our Bodies, Ourselves *Revised Edition*
Boston Women's Health Book Collective
Written by women, for women, to help them know themselves and their bodies better. Covers sexuality, contraception, women and health care, sexual physiology, and reproduction. *Simon & Schuster (1976), 1230 Avenue of the Americas, New York, N.Y. 10020.*

Our Right to Love: A Lesbian Resource Book
Ginny Vida, ed.
Sensitively chosen, remarkable collection of essays written by and for lesbians about their needs and values. *Prentice-Hall (1978), Englewood Cliffs, N.J. 07632.*

Shared Intimacies
Lonnie Barbach and Linda Levine
Descriptions of women's positive sexual experiences and their inventive solutions to sexual problems, thus providing a way for women to learn from one another. *Doubleday (1980), 501 Franklin Ave., Garden City, N.Y. 11530. Bantam, 666 Fifth Ave., New York, N.Y. 10019.*

Womancare: A Gynecological Guide to Your Body
Linda Madaras and Jane Patterson
A comprehensive text of obstetrics and gynecology written for laypersons, especially women. *Avon (1981), 959 Eighth Ave., New York, N.Y. 10019.*

Woman's Body: An Owner's Manual
The Diagram Group
Well-illustrated guide with clear, straightforward information for women of all ages. *Bantam (1978), 666 Fifth Ave., New York, N.Y. 10019.*

Women: Menopause and Middle Age
Vidal S. Clay
A moving, compassionate book that contributes to a positive recognition of the right of postmenopausal women to a full sexual life. Includes a useful annotated bibliography and several self-study exercises. *Know (1977), Box 86031, Pittsburgh, Pa. 15221.*

FOR MEN AND WOMEN

Abortion to Zoophilia: A Sourcebook of Sexual Facts
Anne Mandetta and Patricia Gustaveson
A clear, sensible, information-packed book of sexual facts, conveniently presented and backed with references. Contains a 520-item index. *Carolina Population Center (1976), Educational Materials Unit, University Sq. 300 A, Chapel Hill, N.C. 27514.*

Changing Views of Homosexuality *Public Affairs Pamphlet #563*
Elizabeth Ogg
Written in nontechnical language. Public Affairs pamphlets are known for covering their subject matter in a concise, effective manner. *Public Affairs Committee (1978), 381 Park Ave. South, New York, N.Y. 10016.*

A Child Is Born *Revised Edition*
Mirjam Furuhjelm, Axel Ingelman-Sundberg, and Claes Wirsen
Provides detailed description of fetal development, illustrated by the famous Lennart Nilsson photographs. Useful for explaining reproduction to groups from adolescents through expectant parents. *Delacorte (1977), 1 Dag Hammarskjold Plaza, New York, N.Y. 10017.*

A Disturbed Peace: Selected Writings of an Irish-Catholic Homosexual
Brian McNaught
Unique and revealing autobiography in the form of a collection of essays written over several years. Could serve as an excellent introduction to homosexuality for heterosexual people. *Dignity (1981), 1500 Massachusetts Ave., N.W., Washington, D.C. 20005.*

The Joy of Sex: A Gourmet Guide to Lovemaking
Alex Comfort
A finely illustrated, civilized, and explicit guide to lovemaking. *Simon & Schuster (1974), 1230 Avenue of the Americas, New York, N.Y. 10020.*

Learning to Love: How to Make Bad Sex Good and Good Sex Better
Paul Brown and Carolyn Faulder
A subtle and valuable combination of sexual information, clearly described exercises, case histories, and permission-giving attitudes. *Universe (1978), 381 Park Ave. South, New York, N.Y. 10016.*

Making Love During Pregnancy
Elizabeth Bing and Libby Colman
Frank, firsthand description of pregnancy experiences. Discusses fears and misconceptions of future parents. *Bantam (1977), 666 Fifth Ave., New York, N.Y. 10019.*

More Joy
Alex Comfort
A sequel to *The Joy of Sex*, emphasizing the role of sex in improving relationships and personal growth. Includes sections on sex and aging, and sex and the disabled. Also discusses less conventional sex styles such as group sex. *Simon & Schuster (1975), 1230 Avenue of the Americas, New York, N.Y. 10020.*

Questions and Answers About Love and Sex
Mary S. Calderone and the editors of* Bride's *magazine
Excellent practical guide and reference source. Encourages the development of healthy sexual attitudes in marital relationships. *St. Martin's (1979), 175 Fifth Ave., New York, N.Y. 10010.*

SAR Guide for a Better Sex Life
National Sex Forum
A provocative manual for persons interested in examining their sexual attitudes and practices in order to enrich their experiences and stimulate new perspectives. *Multi Media Resources Center (1977), 1525 Franklin St., San Francisco, Calif. 94109.*

The Sex Atlas: New Popular Reference Edition
Erwin J. Haeberle
A comprehensive sourcebook of basic textual information on human sexuality. *Continuum (1982), 575 Lexington Ave., New York, N.Y. 10022.*

Sex Facts
A simply written booklet for *all* ages—anyone over 12. Discusses sex and sexuality, birth control, orgasm, sex problems, and much more. *Planned Parenthood of Syracuse (1977), 1120 East Genesee St., Syracuse, N.Y. 13210.*

Sex Talk
Myron Brenton
Recognizing the need for clear communication about sex between man and woman, parent and child, suggests how such communication can be achieved. *Stein & Day (1977), Scarborough House, Briarcliff Manor, N.Y. 10510.*

Sex: The Facts, the Acts, and Your Feelings
Michael Carrera
Comprehensive, accurate, and easy-to-understand information about sexuality presented in a nonjudgmental tone, imparting values concerned with people and relationships. Also useful for adolescents. *Crown (1981), 1 Park Ave., New York, N.Y. 10016.*

Sexual Myths and Fallacies
James Leslie McCary
Seventy sexual myths explored in the light of the best information available. *Schocken (1973), 200 Madison Ave., New York, N.Y. 10016.*

*

Parents

The Family Book About Sexuality
Mary S. Calderone and Eric W. Johnson
A creative, comprehensive approach to a family's understanding of the sexuality and sexual concerns of all its members. Includes encyclopedic glossary of terms. *Harper & Row (1981), 10 East 53rd St., New York, N.Y. 10022. Bantam, 666 Fifth Ave., New York, N.Y. 10019.*

A Family Matter: A Parents' Guide to Homosexuality
Charles Silverstein
Written for parents with a homosexual child, examining the realities of the situation and suggesting how to turn the experience into a positive relationship. *McGraw-Hill (1977), 1221 Avenue of the Americas, New York, N.Y. 10020.*

Growing Up Free: Raising Your Child in the '80s
Letty Cottin Pogrebin
Covers child rearing from conception to maturity. Emphasizes nonsexist sex education, parity parenting, and gender-neutral attitudes. Highly recommended. *McGraw-Hill (1980), 1221 Avenue of the Americas, New York, N.Y. 10020. Bantam (1981), 666 Fifth Ave., New York, N.Y. 10019.*

Not My Daughter: Facing Up to Adolescent Pregnancy
Katherine B. Oettinger with Elizabeth Mooney
Helpful for parents and for those seeking perspectives on the problem in their search for preventive measures. Stresses need for early communication between adults and teens. *Prentice-Hall (1979), Englewood Cliffs, N.J. 07632.*

Now That You Know: What Every Parent Should Know About Homosexuality
Betty Fairchild and Nancy Hayward
Informative, sensitively written guide for parents of homosexuals. Highly recommended. *Harcourt Brace Jovanovich (1979), 757 Third Ave., New York, N.Y. 10017.*

Oh No! What Do I Do Now?
Handling Children's Behavior and Answering Children's Questions
CHOICE and SIECUS
A simply written pamphlet which describes an approach for parents of children under six to use in determining possible responses to eight situations and questions commonly encountered. Available also in Spanish. *SIECUS (1981), 80 Fifth Ave., Suite 801, New York, N.Y. 10011.*

On Becoming a Family: The Growth of Attachment
T. Berry Brazelton
Provides reassuring and meaningful support for parents-to-be and, step by step, beginning with the earliest moment of awareness of pregnancy, leads to a full understanding of the growth of a family. *Delta (1981), 1 Dag Hammarskjold Plaza, New York, N.Y. 10017.*

The Parent's Guide to Teenage Sex and Pregnancy
Howard R. Lewis and Martha E. Lewis
Dealing mainly with teenage intercourse and its ramifications, this practical book tells parents how to talk to children about sex in ways youngsters understand and accept; how to help teenagers resist peer pressures toward premature intercourse; which birth control methods to recommend (without encouraging intercourse); and, if a daughter or a son's girlfriend should get pregnant, what considerations are important in weighing abortion, adoption, keeping the baby, and marriage. *Berkley (1982), 200 Madison Ave., New York, N.Y. 10016. St. Martin's (1980), 175 Fifth Ave., New York, N.Y. 10010.*

Right from the Start: A Guide to Non-Sexist Childrearing
Selma Greenberg
Recommended for parents who want to help children of either sex build on their own particular strengths. Redefines motherhood, fatherhood, and family power relationships and demonstrates how differential treatment of boys and girls hinders their development. *Houghton Mifflin (1979), 1 Beacon St., Boston, Mass. 02107.*

Schools and Parents—Partners in Sex Education *Public Affairs Pamphlet #581*
Sex Education: The Parents' Role *Public Affairs Pamphlet #549*
Sol Gordon and Irving R. Dickman
Well-written pamphlets designed to give advice and accurate information to parents. *Public Affairs Committee (1980, 1977), 381 Park Ave. South, New York, N.Y. 10016.*

Sex Education Begins at Home: How to Raise Sexually Healthy Children
Howard R. Lewis and Martha E. Lewis
Primarily directed at parents of children through the early teens, this practical guide gives tips on handling sexual discussions; providing a model of healthy sexuality; dealing with problems in emotional and physical development; beating the dating game; and addressing such sensitive issues as masturbation and same-sex experimentation. *Appleton-Century-Crofts (1983), 25 Van Zant St., East Norwalk, Conn. 06855.*

Talking with Your Child About Sex
Mary S. Calderone and James W. Ramey
Random House (1983), 201 East 50th St., New York, N.Y. 10022.

Teenage Pregnancy: What Can Be Done? *Public Affairs Pamphlet #594*
Irving R. Dickman
A concise analysis of the problem. *Public Affairs Committee (1981), 381 Park Ave. South, New York, N.Y. 10016.*

Why Is That Lady's Tummy So Big?
CHOICE
Booklet to help parents answer young children's questions about sex. *CHOICE (1981), 1501 Cherry St., Philadelphia, Pa. 19102.*

Winning the Battle for Sex Education
Irving R. Dickman
Designed to help parents, teachers, administrators, and other members of a community effectively organize support for a public school sex education program. Includes answers to the 20 questions most often asked about such programs. *SIECUS (1982), 80 Fifth Ave., Suite 801, New York, N.Y. 10011.*

*

Older Adults

The Fires of Autumn: Sexual Activity in the Middle and Later Years
Peter A. Dickinson
Encyclopedic and wide open on the topic of sexuality and aging. Written in a witty and humorous style. *Sterling (1977), 2 Park Ave., New York, N.Y. 10016.*

Good Sex After Fifty
Ruth K. Witkin and Robert J. Nissen
Compact, well-written booklet designed to encourage middle-aged and older people to maintain their sexual life. *Regency (1980), 32 Ridge Dr., Port Washington, N.Y. 11050.*

Love and Sex After Sixty: A Guide for Men and Women for Their Later Years
Robert N. Butler and Myrna I. Lewis
A practical book giving older people guidance in enjoying—to whatever degree and in whatever way they wish—the satisfactions of physical sex and pleasurable sensuality. *Harper & Row (1977), 10 East 53rd St., New York, N.Y. 10022.*

Sex After Sixty-Five *Public Affairs Pamphlet #519*
Norman M. Lobsenz
A useful overview of sexuality in the later years. *Public Affairs Committee (1975), 381 Park Ave. South, New York, N.Y. 10016.*

Sexuality and Aging
Mona Wasow
Sensitively written booklet for older people, maintaining that sex should be a pleasure, not a bore. Large print for easy reading. *Family Life (1976), 219 Henderson St., P.O. Box 427, Saluda, N.C. 28773.*